ETHICAL ISSUES IN RESEARCH

ETHICAL ISSUES
IN RESEARCH

Edited by

Darwin Cheney

University Publishing Group, Inc.
Frederick, Maryland 21701

ISBN 1-55572-016-1

Table of Contents

PART IV
USE OF EMBRYOS AND FETUSES

PART V
USE OF ANIMALS

PART IV

Contributors

Paul J. Anderson, MD, is the editor of the *Journal of Histochemistry and Cytochemistry,* Mount Sinai School of Medicine, City University of New York.

Zbigniew Bankowski, MD, is Secretary General of the Council for International Organizations of Medical Sciences (CIOMS), Geneva, Switzerland.

Sharon G. Boots, PhD, is Chair of the Editorial Policy Committee, Council of Biology Editors, Inc.; and Managing Editor of *Analytical Chemistry,* the American Chemical Society, Washington, DC.

James Bopp, Jr., JD, is a member of the NIH Fetal Tissue Transplant Panel; and a member of the law firm of Bopp, Coleson, and Bostrom, Terre Haute, Indiana.

Addeane S. Caelleigh is the editor of *Academic Medicine,* Association of American Medical Colleges, Washington, DC.

Darwin L. Cheney, PhD, is Director of the Fidia Research Foundation, Washington, DC.

Albin Eser, MCJ, is Professor and Director of the Max-Planck-Institute for Foreign and International Criminal Law; and Vice President of the German Research Foundation, Bonn.

Paul J. Friedman, MD, is Professor and Dean for Academic Affairs at the School of Medicine, University of California-San Diego, La Jolla.

Clifford Grobstein, PhD, is Professor Emeritus of Biological Science at the University of California-San Diego, La Jolla.

Suzanne W. Hadley, PhD, is Deputy Director of the Office of Scientific Integrity at the National Institutes of Health, Bethesda, Maryland.

Jules V. Hallum, PhD, is Director of the Office of Scientific Integrity at the National Institutes of Health, Bethesda, Maryland.

Barbara C. Hansen, PhD, is Professor of Physiology and Director of the Obesity and Diabetes Research Center at the University of Maryland School of Medicine, Baltimore.

Kenneth D. Hansen, MD, JD, is a Professor at the University of Maryland School of Medicine, Baltimore.

Raymond Hoffenberg, MD, PhD, FRCP, is President of Wolfson College, Oxford, England.

Edward J. Huth, MD, is the editor of *Online Journal of Current Clinical Trials;* and is Editor Emeritus and book review editor of *Annals of Internal Medicine.*

David Korn, MD, is Vice President and Dean of Stanford University School of Medicine, Stanford, California.

T. David Marshall, MD, LLB, LMCC, JSC, is a Justice of the Ontario Court of Justice, General Division, Hamilton; a Justice of the Supreme Court and Court of Appeals of the Northwest Territories and Yukon Territories; and Chairman of the Standing Committee on Ethics and Human Experimentation, Medical Research Council of Canada.

M.J. Matfield, PhD, is a member of the Research Defence Society, London, England.

Allan Mazur, PhD, is a Professor of Public Affairs at the Maxwell School, Syracuse University, New York.

Barbara Mishkin, MA, JD, is an attorney specializing in health-regulatory issues at the law firm of Hogan & Hartson, Washington, DC.

William B. Neaves, PhD, is a Professor of Cell Biology and Dean of the Southwestern Medical Center, University of Texas, Dallas.

Roger J. Porter, MD, is Vice President of Clinical Research at Wyeth-Ayerst Laboratories, Radnor, Pennsylvania.

Vittorio Sgaramella, PhD, is Professor of Molecular Biology in the Department of Genetics and Microbiology, University of Pavia, Italy.

Adil E. Shamoo, PhD, is a member of the Center for Biomedical Ethics, and a research biochemist at the Department of Biological Chemistry, University of Maryland School of Medicine, Baltimore.

Kern Wildenthal, MD, PhD, is a Professor of Physiology and Internal Medicine and Dean of the Southwestern Medical Center, University of Texas, Dallas.

Patricia K. Woolf, PhD, is Professor of Microbiology at the Lewis Thomas Laboratory, Department of Microbiology.

Ethics in Research: An Overview

Darwin L. Cheney

Today, it is almost impossible to pick up a scientific journal without seeing another charge or countercharge of scientific misconduct. Even more disheartening is to see those same charges appearing with increasing frequency in the popular press. Maintenance of high ethical standards in research is absolutely essential if we are to maximize the benefits of health-related scientific discoveries to the general population. To settle for anything less will mean a squandering of the meager resources available to the scientific community.

A basic tenet of scientific inquiry is to elucidate "truth." Research colleagues depend on "truthful" reporting of scientific results even if they would challenge the interpretation. Health-care providers depend on "truthfully" reported clinical trials to properly treat disease. Unethical conduct destroys the fabric of "truth" and causes researchers to waste precious time and money. The apparent loss of integrity among seekers of truth may well erode public confidence in scientific research and further reduce vital research dollars.

This volume deals with several ethical issues: (1) How can the scientific community appropriately respond to instances of deliberate misrepresentation of data in its many forms? (2) How can the scientific community prevent the conflict of interest that appears to be inherent in the commercialism of scientific discoveries? (3) How can the scientific community respond to external pressures that would prevent the use of human subjects, embryos and fetuses, or animals in research?

The authors of the various chapters have examined the role of academic, institutional, and governmental research centers in promoting responsible conduct of research. They have identified major issues facing researchers; they have identified areas in which progress has been made; and they have recommended actions that may be undertaken to resolve some of these complex issues. This compilation of views, opinions, and suggestions may help to raise the awareness of scientists and administrators to enable them to prevent scientific misconduct, to provide guidelines to handle incidents of misconduct appropriately, and to respond appropriately to external pressures.

HOW CAN THE SCIENTIFIC COMMUNITY RESPOND TO INSTANCES OF DELIBERATE MISREPRESENTATION OF DATA?

Hallum and Hadley in their chapter, "Office of Scientific Integrity: Why, What, and How," state that there must be a partnership among the scientific researchers, the institutes and universities, and government "watchdog" agencies to "reestablish the high regard of science by the public and its representatives." These same entities (researchers, institutes/ universities, and government agencies) have important and overlapping responsibilities to expose incidents of scientific misconduct in order to maintain high ethical standards in research.

In her chapter, "Distinguishing Between Error and Fraud," Woolf argues that peer review is the major quality-control mechanism in judging science and that the whole scientific enterprise is designed to eliminate error. When scientists are not sufficiently "scrupulous in correcting important errors and in making clear distinctions between honest errors and fraud," the bonds of trust among investigators are weakened and the self-regulating system is impaired. Unfortunately, those who are most competent to judge between honest errors and fraud "have an interest in minimizing the impact of that judgment on their institutions and on public perceptions of science," according to Friedman in his chapter "Misrepresentation of Data and the Integrity of Research: Many Perspectives." He concludes that while this is a serious conflict of interest, it is best resolved by "disclosure and discussion" within the institution and not by relegating these problems to the adversarial environment of the courts or abdicating responsibility to a federal agency.

There is little disagreement that institutions that support scientific research have an obligation to resolve instances of scientific misconduct; indeed, a number of universities, professional organizations, and federal governmental bodies have developed procedures for handling allegations of scientific misconduct. In the chapter entitled "Treatment of Allegations of Research Misconduct by American Universities," Mazur outlines general procedures by which universities may deal with allegations of misconduct. He then uses these procedures as a model to evaluate how universities have responded to allegations of fraud or misconduct by members of their staff.

In order to ensure that institutions receiving public funds have policies and procedures in place to deal with alleged or suspected scientific misconduct, in 1989 the Public Health Service established the Office of Scientific Integrity

(OSI) and the Office of Scientific Integrity Review (OSIR). More recently, these two independent but complementary entities have been renamed the Division of Research Integrity Assurance and the Division of Policy, respectively, and have been combined under the Office of Research Integrity. These governmental agencies oversee the implementation of all policies and procedures related to matters of possible scientific misconduct; oversee each investigation into alleged or suspected scientific misconduct by any institution applying for or receiving PHS research funds; conduct inquiries or investigations, when necessary; and participate in and direct preventative and educational measures to encourage the responsible conduct of research. The ultimate purpose of these functional interrelationships among governmental entities, institutes, and universities, and members of the scientific community is to restore the public trust that appears to have been eroded over the past few years.

Various terms have been used to categorize the seriousness of scientific misconduct and the practices by which data may be altered for more favorable presentation. Woolf and Friedman have discussed them in some detail in their respective chapters. With the advent of computer imagery, another type of misrepresentation of data is creeping into the scientific literature--manipulation of computer images in scientific documentation. Anderson discusses the full ramifications of computer-generated alterations in some detail in the chapter entitled "Authorship and Illustrations: The Challenge of Computer Manipulation." Computer-stored images are easily manipulated to add or subtract details, modify colors, or combine subject matter from several sources. These computer adjustments are undetectable and are rarely documented. Anderson recommends that organizations concerned with publication standards should address the need for guidelines in the use of computer-generated or "edited" graphics.

Authorship in science is an ill-defined term and is fraught with abuses. Scientific journal editors (Boots, Editor, *Analytical Chemistry*; Caelleigh, Editor, *Academic Medicine*; Huth, Editor Emeritus, *Annals of Internal Medicine*) contend that in an environment where publications have come to play a key role in raises, tenure, and promotion, pressures to publish create conditions in which more names are added as authors and the published unit (that is, the amount of original information presented) becomes smaller. Caelleigh, in her chapter "Taking Responsibility as an Author," reviews the guidelines written by the International Committee of Medical Journal Editors; and Huth, in his chapter "Should Scientific Authorship be Controlled?" reviews the guidelines written by the Council of Biology Editors. Guidelines such as these, need to be drafted by all journals to enable researchers to answer the questions of who should be responsible and who should receive public credit for the work reported in the article. Boots stresses in her chapter "Is Being an Author the Key to Success?" that to further reduce abuses associated with authorship, universities and granting agencies should reduce the importance placed on numbers of publications for raises, tenure, promotions, and grant renewals.

Scientific misconduct is not a phenomenon that is limited to the United States. Eser (Germany), Sgaramella (Italy), and Hoffenberg (United Kingdom) in their chapters, respectively entitled "Misrepresentation of Data and Other Misconduct in Science: German View and Experience," "The Recombinant DNA Revolution and the Concept of Pure Research in Biomedical Sciences," and "Fraud in Medicine: Its Causes and Control--A UK View," clearly indicate that while scientific misconduct has not had the public focus in other countries of the world, the problem is international.

HOW CAN THE SCIENTIFIC COMMUNITY PREVENT CONFLICT OF INTEREST IN THE COMMERCIALISM OF SCIENTIFIC DISCOVERIES?

Mishkin, in her chapter "Cooperation Between Academia and Industry: Opportunities and Challenges," describes an area of scientific misconduct that has received considerable attention as scientists, institutes/universities, and governmental agencies try to grapple with its implications. "Conflict of interest," in the scientific community, as defined by Korn, in his chapter "Conflict of Interest: A University Perspective," refers to "situations in which financial or other personal considerations may compromise, or have the appearance of compromising, a physician's professional judgement in delivering patient care, or an investigator's professional judgement in conducting or reporting research."

Conflict of interest is a function of the motives of the scientist and not the science that is produced. Porter, in his chapter "Scientific Motivation and Conflicts of Interest in Research," purports that the wrong motivation may temporarily distort the accuracy of scientific findings or delay their communication, but truth will eventually prevail. In the process of commercialization of biomedical science, investigators have had to face the ethical dilemma of assuming such confusing roles as entrepreneurs, research scientists, and educators all at once. Hansen and Hansen, in their chapter "Managing Conflict of Interest in Faculty, Federal Government and Industrial Relations," evaluate the varied roles of the scientist, the institution, and the government in the commercialization of a research discovery. Neaves and Wildenthal, in their chapter "Conflict of Interest Issues Surrounding Faculty Participation in, and Ownership of, Technology and Drug Companies," deal with issues that have arisen at the University of Texas Southwestern Medical Center during the development and implementation of a new technology transfer program. Both chapters conclude that full disclosure of all financial and consultatory relationships is a primary requisite, but is not sufficient. Guidelines have been formulated by the Association of Academic Health Centers and the Association of American Medical Colleges to assist in dealing with faculty conflicts of interest and are referenced by Neaves and Wildenthal. In addition, NIH has proposed guidelines, which have not yet been implemented, for academic institutions to follow in dealing with this thorny issue.

Shamoo, in his chapter entitled "Role of Conflict of Interest in Public Advisory Councils," points out the potential for conflict of interest inherent among those who serve on advisory councils, advisory boards, study sections, and review panels for government-granting agencies. The experts who are asked to serve must have sufficient expertise within the narrow professional field to make fair judgments as they evaluate grant applications, and these same experts may well be competing for the same pool of funds. In order to minimize the potential for conflict of interest, Shamoo recommends that whenever possible "direct competitors" should not serve on advisory groups. However, when a direct competitor's expertise is absolutely necessary for an advisory group, his or her conflict of interest should be clearly stated.

HOW CAN THE SCIENTIFIC COMMUNITY RESPOND TO EXTERNAL PRESSURES CONCERNING THE USE OF HUMAN SUBJECTS, EMBRYOS AND FETUSES, OR ANIMALS IN RESEARCH?

Use of Human Subjects in Research

Bankowski, in his chapter "International Ethical Guidelines for Research on Human Subjects," stresses the importance of international ethical guidelines for research on human subjects. The Nuremberg Code and the Declaration of Helsinki provide ethical guidelines for research involving human subjects. Because of the potential for exploitation of communities within developing countries, the Council for International Organizations of medical Sciences (CIOMS) and the World Health Organization (WHO) issued their Proposed International Guidelines for Biomedical Research Involving Human Subjects. International guidelines must be very general to satisfy all countries and cultures; consequently, there must be active involvement of scientists, health professionals, philosophers, lawyers, and theologians to ensure that the guidelines protect all people everywhere and to ensure that biomedical and epidemiological research benefits all of humanity.

Use of Human Fetal Tissue in Research

Important ethical issues are involved in the uses of early human developmental stages in research. Although there is little disagreement within the general community that research using human fetal tissue has the potential of providing great benefit in the treatment of a number of human disorders, some would argue that the ethical considerations against using fetal tissue outweigh these potential benefits. As noted above with the treatment of human subjects of research, related ethical issues of comparable difficulty have been addressed and guidelines put in place that appear to function successfully. It is now imperative that the ethical issues involved in the uses of fetal tissue in research be given careful consideration and resolved. This will not be an easy task. The government has placed a moratorium on human development research that it once funded. Moreover, the potential relationships between research facilities and abortion clinics create entanglements that remain unresolved by either political or ethical arguments.

Grobstein, in his chapter "The Status and Uses of Early Human Development Stages," focuses on the moral and legal status of early human developmental stages and how they should be treated in laboratories and in clinical practice. He contends that "under appropriate oversight and with suitable safeguards, early human developmental stages should be available to gain otherwise unobtainable important new knowledge." Bopp, on the other hand, in his chapter "Ethical Limitations on Use of the Human Fetus in Research," argues that the risk of promoting abortion by using fetal tissue from induced abortions for transplants is too great to make induced abortions ethically acceptable. He contends, therefore, that the federal government policy of not funding fetal transplantation research is justified. Furthermore, if some transplantation research using tissue from induced abortions could be ethically justified, there would still be insufficient federal legislative safeguards to make them ethically acceptable.

The ethical issues alluded to above must not be trivialized or oversimplified by those who would resolve them. The same kind of deliberative approach that now governs the use of adult human beings in research must be extended to the use, in research, of the fetal stages of development.

Use of Animals in Biomedical Research

As society changes from one that is predominately rural to one that is predominantly urban, ethical and legal norms in animal experimentation are altered. Animal rights and animal welfare groups have challenged the treatment and use of animals in biomedical research. Animal welfare groups want assurances that research animals are treated humanely, but are not necessarily opposed to using animals in biomedical research. Animal rights groups maintain that all sentient beings share the same intrinsic rights, and human beings have no special rights to themselves; consequently, any use of animals by humans is immoral or unethical.

The scientific research community has responded by improving the treatment of research animals. The US Department of Agriculture issued its updated rules for care and handling of laboratory animals in February 1991.[1] Processes have been implemented to ensure that animals used in research are treated in accordance with generally accepted principles and laws. Marshall, in his chapter "Evolving Ethical and Legal Norms in Animal Experimentation," discusses the progress that has been made in Canada. Canada has organized local Animal Research Ethics Boards. These boards are composed of scientific members, lay members, specialists in animal husbandry, and specialists in the use of animals in research. To oversee the functioning of these local committees, a Canadian Council on Animal Care has been organized at the national level, which regularly visits institutions and reviews local procedures, with power to order improvements.

Attempts to reduce the number of research animals used in experimentation and attempts to improve research animal care have not been viewed as sufficient by animal rights proponents. There continue to be numerous attempts to limit or abolish experimentation with animals. In fact, in recent years, animal rights organizations have become more violent and extreme. Matfield describes the UK experience in his chapter, "Research and the Response from the Scientific and Medical Community," and indicates that outright terrorist activities by the animal rights movements are far more frequent in Great Britain than any other country. In response to the extreme and violent actions of those who oppose animal research, scientists have begun to fight back and to speak out. Organizations like the Foundation for Biomedical Research and the Research Defence Society in Great Britain have ensured that the scientist's point of view is conveyed to the public using newspapers and television. Organizations like the National Academy of Sciences and Institute of Medicine[2] and the American Medical Association[3] in the United States have published position papers defending the use of animals in research. Department of Health and Human Services Secretary Louis Sullivan has been outspoken in his support of the use of animals in research. He declared publicly that the "so-called animal rights activists" are "nothing more than animal rights terrorists." He added, "they will not succeed, because they are on the wrong side of morality."[4]

Because community norms are changing and will continue to change, it is essential that in every research institution procedures for the ethical and lawful treatment of research animals be established that are impartial, independent of research interests, well informed, representative, and, above all, open. These procedures, according to Marshall, will ensure that "evolving community norms are reflected in decisions and that these decisions are seen by the community as openly arrived at and just."

CONCLUSION

To maintain high ethical standards in research, there must be a partnership among scientific researchers, institutes/universities, and government agencies. There must be active involvement of individual scientists, health professionals, philosophers, lawyers, and theologians to ensure that guidelines are generated and implemented to protect the scientific community and the general public if scientific research is to benefit all of humanity. It is hoped that this compilation of views and opinions of leaders in research, academia, and government will raise the awareness of scientists and administrators to enable them to deal effectively with the various ethical issues discussed herein. Certainly the issue of ethics in research will continue to be a "hot" topic in the future. Approaches must be found to encourage the highest standards of ethical behavior if the pursuit of scientific knowledge in a supportive societal environment is to survive.

NOTES

1   J. Johnston, "USDA Issues Final Dog, Cat, Primate Care Regulations," *Journal of NIH Research* 3 (1991): 43-44.
2   Committee on the Use of Animals in Research, National Academy of Sciences and Institute of Medicine, "Science, Medicine, and Animals," (Washington, DC: National Academy Press, 1991).
3   American Medical Association, *Use of Animals in Biomedical Research: The Challenge and Response*, (Chicago: AMA, 1988).
4   "Secretary Sullivan declares animal activists 'On the wrong side of morality,' " *Public Affairs Newsletter* 23, no.4 (1990): 1.

Part I

Misrepresentation of Data

1

Distinguishing Between Error and Fraud in Science

Patricia K. Woolf

Trustworthy scientific knowledge depends on imaginative, conscientious, and careful attention to the design of experiments and to the collection, interpretation, and reporting of research results. In this process there are innumerable opportunities for errors and self-deception.[1] And, as we have learned in the last generation, there is also opportunity for fraud.[2] Some scientists have deceived their colleagues, their readers, and the public by falsifying, fabricating, or plagiarizing[3] work that they presented as their own honest efforts. And, as a result of the actions of a few and the reactions of many more, questions about the social and political control of science and the resources to be spent on it are being reexamined.

Most people recognize the inevitability of error in human activities and are forgiving, within reason (perhaps because they wish for a parallel indulgence for their own mistakes). Moreover, there are vast social enterprises devoted to preventing, detecting, correcting, compensating for, and undoing the consequences of errors. For instance, there is quality assurance, quality control, modeling and mockups in manufacturing; referees and umpires in sports; internal and external auditing in business and financial activities; review, editing, and proofreading in publishing; and insurance of many kinds, including one called E and O (errors and omissions) for management and directors of public companies. In addition, there is governmental oversight of many of the above. Perhaps even fire departments and the Coast Guard can be considered as backstops for error as well as accident. Wherever there are rules, protocols, or expectations, there will be deviations, and a system for deciding whether or not the variance is acceptable under the terms of the enterprise. Informal estimates for these collective activities to protect against error range from 10 to 20 percent of the US gross national product (GNP).[4] Some of this oversight also protects against poor quality in general, and against deceptive practices including fraud. Error, broadly conceived, is a generally accepted part of life.

But errors in professional activities often raise more ominous issues of negligence. Although it is recognized that there will be mistakes even in the most careful endeavors, the consequences of error--in medical situations for instance --are so dire that an extra burden of care is recognized. Charles Bosk's study of how surgeons learn to cope with error, *Forgive and Remember*, sensitively explores the ways that professionals, individually and collectively, learn from mistakes in order to prevent them in the future.[5] The more dangerous the consequences, the more precautions are taken.

Until recently, however, scientists have enjoyed an important dispensation from the professional requirement to avoid mistakes. The "right to be wrong" is considered to be a privilege of conducting research. And perhaps that may be one mark of the oddity of scientific research as a profession. Within the profession, it is widely believed not only that scientists will inevitably make mistakes in the pursuit of scientific understanding, but also that a slavish attention to minimizing error can actually impair creativity and thereby slow the progress of science.

Errors and mistakes remain part of the craft of science.[6] Doing research requires attempting any number of explorations and distinguishing between those that "work" and those that do not. These views are taken so much for granted that they are rarely discussed: it is a matter of course that scientists will try a lot of experiments that do not work. They will make a lot of observations that turn out to be useless. They will build equipment that malfunctions. Reagents will get stale. Specimens will die. It is not even clear that such failed efforts are errors in the sense that nonscientists think of errors.[7] Similarly, false starts and blind alleys, experiments that misfire, and theories that don't pan out can be regarded--in retrospect--as mistakes or misplaced efforts, but they are not "errors" simply because they turned out to be wrong. They can even be necessary steps toward the "right" answers as they rule out faulty hypotheses.[8] In his study of the concept of fact in science, Fleck states, "Discovery is thus inextricably interwoven with what is known as error. To recognize a certain relation, many another relation must be misunderstood, denied or overlooked.[9] And again, "Error and the failure of many experiments are also part of the building materials for a scientific fact."[10] Research is notoriously inefficient, partly because of the uncertainty about its goals. We know very little, however, about how much erroneous science necessarily accompanies productive and correct research. Should we be comfortable with 50 percent efficiency, or 10 percent, or hold out for 80 or 90 percent?

Attempts to understand scientists' views about error are further compli- cated by the fact that error, in addition to being used loosely as roughly synonymous with mistake, is often used in a strictly technical sense as an intrinsic component of all measurement. Since measurements can never be perfectly precise and accurate, scientists have learned that the deviation (that is, the error) should be quantified, reported, and taken into consideration. But it cannot be eliminated entirely; and, in its technical sense, error can only be reduced. It cannot be "corrected."[11] Indeed, judgment calls about how much measurement error is allowable play a significant role in deciding whether particular data is relevant for making scientific inferences.

It may be that the current turmoil about fraud and error will push scientists toward a refined appreciation of the distinction between this technical use of "error" and other broad categories of errors, mistakes, pratfalls, blunders, gaffes, miscalculations, snafus, misstatements, and mishaps.[12] In the meantime, the following discussion of the concept of error will track general popular usage, and will not be limited to uncertainty in measurement.

If there has been little discussion of the role of errors in research, there has been even less of what constitutes error, and in particular how, when, and if errors--especially those published in the scientific literature--ought to be corrected.[13] Is that because individual articles are not regarded as sufficiently consequential to correct because they are considered only a small part of a self-correcting process? Or is it because the very concept of a mistake depends on an accepted definition of what the desirable outcome ought to be? And that cannot be the case in basic research because the shape and scope of new knowledge is, by its nature, not definable.

In one sense, the whole scientific enterprise is addressed to eliminating error. Although it is widely understood, it is almost never stated that in the pursuit of knowledge, mistakes are useful only to the extent that they are disclosed or generally recognized and, if necessary, corrected. When errors or shortcomings are known, scientists can work within the limitations imposed by that knowledge. Scientists also recognize that on occasion, pursuing an erroneous hypothesis can lead to exciting new ideas and sound results, because researchers are temporarily freed from the constraints of prior theories. But perceptions of when it is "necessary" to correct scientific errors, of whatever sort, are very localized (by discipline and by institution). They are rarely discussed explicitly and are not well understood.

Recent allegations of fraud and misconduct in science are forcing scientists to take the concept of error seriously because the distinction between fraud and error has been blurred in the agitated discussions of what went wrong in several specific cases, and in general. Congressional inquiries, particularly those chaired by Congressman John Dingell, are regarded by many scientists as egregiously offensive in treating what was alleged to be, and thought to be, error as though it were fraud.[14] But, as the various investigations progressed, it became clear that some of the scientists themselves were not sufficiently concerned about acknowledging and correcting errors, and censuring fraud when it occurred. Furthermore, some showed themselves to be reluctant even to retract publications that were demonstrably fraudulent.[15]

Scientists may not have recognized what an extraordinary privilege it is to make mistakes with public monies and to be in charge of determining what is and is not an error. They must be scrupulous in correcting important errors and in making clear distinctions between honest errors and fraud. Policy makers will be more comfortable with the latitude that scientists enjoy when they are sure that scientific specialists within a particular research discipline agree on the criteria for deciding when errors are significant and are seriously committed to continuing quality control.

Two sorts of issues have attracted particular attention as a result of the Congressional concern about research fraud: (1) Is the damage caused by sloppy, negligent, or opportunistic research more significant (because it is more frequent) than the damage caused by putatively rare instances of deceptive or fraudulent research? A related issue concerns deliberate deception short of lying, such as failure to tell everything that scientists need to know in order to evaluate published research.[16] (2) As a matter of policy, what should be done to resolve difficulties with research when it is not clear whether they have been caused by error, by fraud, or by poor professional judgment? And who should take the responsibility for doing so?

I believe that in science the risks associated with fraud and deliberate deception are far greater than those associated with error. Even if fraud is less frequent than error, it is more consequential. Even if the empirical deviation (the magnitude of the discrepancy between presented data and the accurate or "true" situation) is the same, fraud is more consequential. Even if the answer obtained by fraudulent means is "right" (that is, it agrees with the current orthodoxy), a deceptive practice is more consequential because it is destructive to science and to scientists. The basis for this belief is that scientific research consists of its processes as well as its products. Scientific research cannot and should not stand or fall on the accuracy of its product alone: the currently acceptable view of the natural world. It is an "enormously complex system of activities that deliver what counts, at least for the time being, as 'knowledge.' "[17] The current view is always provisional, always subject to correction or improvement in the light of new information; today's version is today's best approximation to understanding. The strength of science lies in its process: the flexibility and the impulse to revise, to correct, and to improve. Allegations of fraud and institutional mishandling of charges have challenged the ability and the desire of scientists to keep the processes of revision vigorous, fair, and open, and have called into question the effectiveness of quality-control mechanisms in research. They thus impair the ability of scientists to trust each other as they work separately and together on common problems.

O'TOOLE AND IMANISHI-KARI

The initial charge by Margot O'Toole in the "Baltimore" case concerned what were called "errors" in the work of Imanishi-Kari published in 1986.[18] O'Toole first presented her concerns to the coauthors, then to university authorities at MIT and Tufts. But as the allegations and the responses of MIT and Tufts University were discussed in seminars and meetings around the country, there was considerable innuendo: although the word "error" was used, the implied charge was one of potential misconduct. Some who heard these seminars notified the coauthors. Prior to the Congressional hearing on 12 April 1988, one of Congressman John Dingell's staff was quoted in the *Boston Globe*[19] as saying, "It's hard to tell if it's error or fraud. At certain times it appears to be fraud and other times misrepresentation."

Dr. O'Toole, who made the initial allegations against Dr. Imanishi-Kari's work, testified about "discrepancies," "error," and "serious inaccuracies."[20] Witness Charles Maplethorpe, a former student in Dr. Imanishi-Kari's laboratory, answered "yes" to a direct question whether he "had observed what [he] felt was falsified and misrepresented data."[21] This was the first explicit accusation of research misconduct that was made public. Scientists--not only the accused authors--were angered that the hearings had apparently escalated an initial charge of error to one of fraud in a situation where the accused scientists (the authors of the Cell paper) and their institutions had no chance to respond in the hearing.[22] But to those others who did not accept the distinction between error and fraud as a matter of profound belief, the accused coauthors had had ample opportunity to respond to O'Toole's charges. Had the coauthors met and together examined all the relevant documents, responding point by point to her criticism (whether of error or fraud), it is doubtful that the issue would have come to such an operatic conclusion.

This situation appeared to be one in which error was alleged and fraud was implied and later charged. University officials could understandably have been in some doubt about a proper course of action, because the consequences of error are often *de minimus* and certainly remain a matter for the judgment of specialists in the field. In a formal sense, the authors and the institutions were only required to respond to the allegation of error. According to the scientific ethos that accepts error as a matter of course, that response need not be as urgent or as draconian as a response to an allegation of fraud.

But the response was insufficient. (In retrospect, it was probably insufficient even for a charge of error.) An error "persisted in" can look like deliberate deception.[23] Paradoxically, it may have been that the coauthors' confidence in the effectiveness of the quality-control mechanisms in science allowed a certain lassitude with regard to the immediate need to correct a specific finding. Scientists who make allegations of error must expect that their charges will be treated differently than allegations of fraud. More recently, the leaked draft report of the National Institutes of Health Office of Scientific Integrity (OSI) noted that Dr. Eisen's memorandum on his review at MIT of O'Toole's allegations was titled "Allegations of misconduct by Thereza Imanishi-Kari. . . ." even though public statements from MIT and Tufts had stated that there had been no formal allegation of fraud.[24] In the light of such subsequent disclosures, if true, the above interpretation may appear charitable, but it is the one that the scientific community thought it had to deal with at the initial unfolding of the case.

Many scientists who read reports of the hearing were disturbed by the situation in which the Cell authors and the research institutions were apparently asked to respond to "errors" and subsequently accused of failing to respond to charges of fraud. They felt that to treat error as if it were fraud would undermine trust and the cooperative practices on which research depends. These scientists and others took it as a matter of faith that they and their colleagues had to be, and were, at ease with the notion of making and correcting errors.

Subsequent developments have shown that they are more comfortable with the notion in principle than in practice. And they are more comfortable with other scientists' corrections than with having to make them themselves. For instance, David Baltimore's letter to Herman Eisen, who conducted the inquiry for MIT (at a time when Baltimore thought there were genuine problems with the research) documents his reluctance to admit and correct errors because he thought "a retraction would harm the innocent [researchers] and raise doubts about quite solid work."[25] Why should publishing a correction harm the innocent if errors are part of the normal work of science? Raising doubts should be commonplace and healthy. Baltimore went on to elaborate a rather typical view about error when he said, "The literature is full of bits and pieces now known to be wrong, but it is not the tradition to point out each one publicly."[26] This letter became a major feature in a subsequent hearing of Mr. Dingell's committee in May 1989. Baltimore forthrightly acknowledged at the hearing that the Cell article should have been corrected.[27] But he did not mention the matter at all in a subsequent article about the controversy in Issues in Science and Technology, published by the National Academy of Sciences.[28] He missed an opportunity to acknowledge the difference between the ideal and the actual, and to urge his colleagues to become more comfortable with correcting errors when it is called for.

ERRORS AND MISTAKES: WHAT DO WE KNOW ABOUT THEM?

Further evidence for the discomfort associated with error and corrections is that so little is known or taught about errors; for instance, how they arise, what research is most susceptible, how to avoid them, how to detect them, when to correct them, how to pick up errors in review, and how to read published articles critically. Is the concept of error so elusive or so discipline-specific that nothing serious can be said about it? Its importance in the ideology of scientific research requires that conflicting uses of the concept be reconciled.

Students learn about Type 1 and Type 2 error in methods or in statistics courses, but I believe those lessons are less frequently associated with practical tasks of assessing research. Although psychologists study experimenter effects, it is not clear that other scientists acknowledge that work as relevant to their own experience. They should be taught to recognize how frequently errors occur. They should know their own susceptibility to error, including that it is not a shameful matter to make mistakes--especially if you catch them on your own.

Rosenthal's (1978) summary of 21 studies in which over 300 persons made 140,000 observations in psychological studies suggested an error rate of about 1 percent with approximately two-thirds of the errors favoring the hypothesis of the observer.[29] Roth's study showed that "hired-hand research" in sociological surveys is fraught with difficulties, and those lessons could be valuable for many other disciplines.[30] Are hired research assistants more or less careful because they are more dispassionate with regard to anticipated outcomes of research? Or are all junior people susceptible to suggestion and, hence, to bias? What studies have been done concerning laboratory errors? More explicit attention to the social and psychological aspects of conducting research could raise awareness about the frequency and significance of errors, and help to avoid the ones that are consequential.

CORRECTING THE RECORD

Most journals do not have explicit guidelines or policies for retractions of publication or for corrections.[31] The International Committee of Medical Journal Editors (also know as the Vancouver Group) has issued a statement or retraction of research findings for articles that have been determined to be untrustworthy.[32] Although many journals publish errata and corrections, many of those that are published correct typos, missing initials, and errors introduced in publication along with some clearly "material" corrections by the original authors. (*Nature* and *Science* typically publish one to three per issue.) Letters to the editor also address errors that readers have detected.

At present, there is no general agreement about the differences between retraction and correction. Who should take responsibility for defining what sorts of errors should be corrected? It is clearly not a matter only for the authors. Should retractions be limited to (issued only in) cases of fraud? Are retractions appropriate when an article is determined to be invalid for innocent reasons? Does a retraction connote culpability? Should corrections and retractions be peer reviewed? The Vancouver Group recommends that retractions be titled as such, on numbered pages, appear in the table of contents, and be indexed. How can editors encourage appropriate correction of published articles? Many scientists feel that correcting the literature should be easy and relatively free of penalties in the interest of others working in the field.

There are at least three categories of discrepancies that may require attention: fraud, errors and mistakes that should be corrected, and errors that can safely be ignored (which may not be synonymous with numerically small or "harmless"). In theory, community judgments by scientific disciplines determine when an error is too trivial to be worth correcting, when a letter to the editor will suffice, when a correction or retraction is warranted, and when an error is significant enough to write an entire paper to rebut it. But at present those standards are not clear to the public that supports research, nor to the legislators who oversee funding agencies. It may be that with the rapid growth of science and the increasing number of specialties that converge in specific research projects, standards are less and less clear, even to scientists who are the authors of scientific publications.

Secondary retrieval sources for the scientific literature, such as computer databases (BIOSIS, MEDLINE), *Chemical Abstracts*, and the *Science Citation Index*, have grappled with how best to handle corrections, errata, retractions, and comments.[33] But they are dependent on how scientists and journal editors publish these items. Since published corrections often deal with matters that appear to be trivial, it is worthwhile to ponder how scientists and editors decide which errors deserve explicit attention and which can be left to the normal processes of research. For understandable psychological reasons, scientists and journal editors may be less reluctant to publish corrections about trivia than about important matters where the corrections are needed most.

It has also been noted that errors persist in textbooks even after they have been corrected in the journal literature. Many psychology texts included Cyril Burt's data about the heritability of intelligence long after it had been discredited.[34] The perpetuation of scientific error, partly due to the commercial aspects of text publication, is a problem for professional scientists. But at present there are no obvious rewards to induce scientists to meet this professional responsibility, and there may be disincentives for publishers to do so.

Although scientists resent the blurring of the distinction between fraud and error when legislators and investigators do it, scientists themselves use a mind-boggling variety of terms to describe violations of research standards. The following terms are only a sample of those that have been used in adjudicating cases of alleged misconduct. The distinctions may matter to those who made them, and even more, perhaps, to their lawyers. But the nonscientific public may find the distinctions sophistic and self-serving.

In approximate order of putative seriousness the terms are: fraud, fabrication, falsification, plagiarism, misdeeds, irregularities, significant irregularities, gross irregularities, misleading and deceptive practices, grossly misleading data, careless assembly of figures, manipulation of data, "fudged" data, sloppy research, misstatement, misrepresentation, unacceptable scientific judgment, serious lapse in scientific judgment, serious departure from acceptable procedure, possible error in classification, serious conceptual errors, flagrant error, error, minor error, inaccuracies, data that might be incorrect, probable overstatement, "anticipatory writing."

Some of these finely honed distinctions seem designed to minimize the seriousness of an offense or to represent the result of negotiations between accusers and accused.[35] Scientists who will, without evidence, defend an accused colleague's acts as unintentional, would not be likely to assert without evidence that the same acts were intentional. While such an assumption of responsible conduct is probably beneficial in ordinary circumstances, professionalism requires a more carefully considered response when serious charges are made.

A better approach to defining significant departure from accepted practices is therefore needed. Some errors must be corrected and others can be disregarded; those that do not deter the efforts of other scientists to replicate or extend the reported research are less likely to need correction. How do scientists (in practice) decide which errors need to be corrected, whether their own or those of someone else? It is clear that standards differ from field to field, from institution to institution, from laboratory to laboratory, and from individual to individual. Little or no formal teaching addresses the detection and correction of one's own errors, or the critical assessment (including discrepancy detection) of the contributions of others. More study is needed.

Bailar's work on statistics and deception in science provides a possible approach to assessing the importance of various sorts of errors.[36] He argues that errors that damage the inferential process of science should be corrected as soon as they are detected. Thus, errors in the methods and results section of scientific articles are significant because they affect readers' ability to evaluate the analysis and conclusions. Errors in analysis are significant when they obscure shortcomings in the data. Errors in the conclusions can be detected by other thoughtful readers (*caveat lector*) and these need only be corrected explicitly when they can result in harm to the public.[37]

Peer review is the major quality-control mechanism of science, and is the process for judging articles for journal publication, presentations at scientific meetings, evaluations of applications for funding, and promotion and tenure appraisals. But the crucial assessment skills needed for peer review are usually learned on the job, and often in circumstances where there are severe time constraints and social pressures. Should there not be some formal instruction in evaluating research and detecting flaws--one's own and that of others?

To return to the notion of professional errors, where the level of precaution depends on the perception of the potential consequences of error: can it be that scientists think the consequences of error in published papers are so trivial that it is a waste of energy and journal space to correct them? Or is it rather that they have so much faith in the self-correcting nature of science that they feel they can safely go onto the next project, confident that others will, in following up, eliminate all but the "right stuff"?

There are rules, protocols, and expectations in science. There will be deviations. The current system for deciding how much variance is acceptable is diverse and tacit, rather than unified and explicit. Some practices that have been accepted are not acceptable. Strict standards can be one part of a vigorous defense of the seriousness and integrity of the research that is done, funded by public monies. These issues require empirical research and reflection by professionals as they face increasing criticism that there is too much trivial research and too many scientists. If research is too trivial to correct, the public may conclude it is too trivial to fund.

ACKNOWLEDGMENT

Thanks are due to John C. Bailar, Barry T. Peterson, Fred Grinnell, and Giles Constable for helpful criticism.

NOTES

1   D.E. Chubin, "Research Malpractice," *Bioscience* 35, no.2 (1985): 80. Reprinted in *Science Off the Pedestal*.

2   W. Broad and N. Wade, *Betrayers of the Truth* (New York, NY: Simon and Schuster, 1982). See also P.K. Woolf, "Deception in Scientific Research," *Jurimetrics Journal* Fall (1988): 69-95; and A. Kohn, *False Prophets*, (Oxford, England: Basil Blackwell, 1986).

3   This chapter will not address plagiarism, but it is worth noting that several persons accused of plagiarism argued that it was a result of error or inadvertence.

4   J. Harding, President, National Life Insurance Co. Informal communication with author, Vermont, February 1991.

5   C.L. Bosk, *Forgive and Remember* (Chicago: University of Chicago Press, 1979), 32-33, 38-40.

6   J.R. Ravetz, *Scientific Knowledge and Its Social Problems* (New York: Oxford University Press, 1971): especially Chapter 3.

7   See H. Zuckerman, "Deviant Behavior and Social Control in Science," in *Deviance and Social Change*, ed. E. Sagarin, (Beverly Hills: Sage Publications, 1977) for her discussion of error and disreputable error; and H. Zuckerman, "Norms and Deviant Behavior in Science," *Science, Technology and Human Values* 9, no.1 (1984): 7-13. See also C.L. Bosk, *Forgive and Remember,* Chapter 2, for his categories of error: (1) technical error, (2) judgmental error, (3) normative error, (4) quasi-normative error.

8   In this context, it is worth noting the recurrent attention given to "publica-

tion bias"; that is, distortion of the record caused by failure to publish negative results. The argument is that negative results are not necessarily less worthy of attention and certainly not *ipso facto* wrong.

9   L. Fleck, *Genesis and Development of a Scientific Fact* (Chicago: University of Chicago Press, 1979), 30.

10   *Ibid.*, 98; B.T. Peterson. Personal communication with the author and comments on this manuscript, 17 May 1991. Dr. Peterson pointed out the distinction between the technical use of error and the common usage that equates error and mistakes.

11   Peterson, Personal communication.

12   H. von Maanen. "Honest Blunders" (letter), *New Scientist* 3 (1991). Dr. von Maanen has requested that scientists send him instances of their own scientific blunders.

13   Two notable exceptions are the clear definition of error in the statistical sense of potential measurement error and the treatment of errors of inference.

14   "Fraud in NIH Grant Programs," Hearing before the Subcommittee on Oversight and Investigations of the HR Committee on Energy and Commerce, 12 April 1988.

15   R.L. Engler, J.W. Covell, P.J. Friedman, *et al.*, "Misrepresentation and Responsibility in Medical Research," *New England Journal of Medicine* 317 (1987): 1383-89; P. Friedman, "Correcting the Literature Following Fraudulent Publication," *Journal of the American Medical Association* 263 (1990): 1416-91; D. Korn, "Scientific Integrity and Scientific Misconduct: The Interface Between Research Institutions and Journals," in *Peer Review in Scientific Publishing* (Chicago: Council of Biology Editors, 1991):205-12.

16   For a refreshing, candid discussion of how scientists ought to present their findings, see Richard Feynman's commencement address to California Institute of Technology graduates, 1974, in R. Feynman, *Surely You're Kidding Mr. Feynman* (New York: Norton, 1985). Cited in *Responsible Science* (Washington, DC: National Academy of Science, 1992).

17   M. Black, "Scientific Neutrality: Between Truth and Irresponsibility," *Encounter* 51 (August 1978): 56-62.

18   D. Weaver, *et al.*, "Altered Repertoire of Endogenous Immunoglobulin Gene Expression in Transgenic Mice Containing a Rearranged *mu* Heavy Chain Gene," *Cell* 45 (1986): 247-59.

19   J. Forman, "A Noted Researcher's Disputed Work Lands in Congress," *Boston Globe*, 11 April 1988, p. 3.

20   M. O'Toole, Testimony provided in the Fraud in NIH Grant Programs Hearing before the Subcommittee on Oversight and Investigations of the House Review Committee on Energy and Commerce on 12 April 1988.

21   C. Maplethorpe, Testimony provided in the Fraud in NIH Grant Programs Hearing before the Subcommittee on Oversight and Investigations of the House Review Committee on Energy and Commerce on 12 April 1988.

22   D. Baltimore, Testimony provided in the Scientific Fraud Hearing before the Subcommittee on Oversight and Investigations of the House Review Committee on Energy and Commerce; B. Davis, "Fraud vs. Error: The Dingelling of Science," *New York Times,* 9 March 1989, p. A20.

23   For a discussion of reporting errors in medicine, see C. Bosk, *Forgive and Remember,* 38-39.

24   Confidential, untitled draft report of the NIH Office of Scientific Integrity, widely circulated and reported in various newspapers in March and April 1991. See for instance, P. Hilts, *New York Times,* 21 March 1991, p. 1.

25   D. Baltimore. Letter to Herman Eisen, 9 September 1986. See also W.E. Leary, "Inquiry to Reopen in Science Dispute," *New York Times,* 30 April 1989, p. 29.

26   D. Baltimore. Letter to Herman Eisen, 9 September 1986. Also quoted in D.P. Hamilton, "White Coats Black Deeds," *Washington Monthly* (April 1990): 25.

27   D. Baltimore. Testimony before Scientific Fraud Hearing.

28   D. Baltimore, "Baltimore's Travels," *Issues in Science and Technology* (Summer 1989):48-54.

29   R. Rosenthal, "How Often Are Our Numbers Wrong?" *American Psychologist* (November 1978):1005-1008.

30   J. Roth, "Hired Hand Research," *American Sociologist* 1 no.4 (1966):190-96.

31   Survey by D.L. Armbruster, S.A. Selig, M.K. Givins, unpublished manuscript presented at Council of Biology Editors meeting, Denver, 6 May 1991.

32   International Committee of Medical Journal Editors, "Guidelines and uniform requirements for manuscripts submitted to Medical Journals," *New England Journal of Medicine* 324 (1991):424-28.

33   L.A. Colianni, S. Kotzin, and N. Selinger, "NLM Handling of Error and Retraction of Publication," *Journal of the American Medical Association* 263 (1990):246-48; L.A. Colianni, "Mince Pie: Thoughts on the Future from the National Library of Medicine," *CBE Views* 12 (1989):13-7; J. Schnepp, BIOSIS. Telephone interview with author, April 1991; N.D. Wright, NLM. Letter to author, 25 January 1991.

34   D.B. Paul, "The Nine Lives of Discredited Data," *The Sciences* (May-June 1987):26-30.

35   For further discussion, see P.K. Woolf, "Accountability and Responsibility in Research," presented at the American Association for the Advancement of Science (AAAS) Annual Meeting, New Orleans, February 1990.

36   J.C. Bailar, "Science Statistics and Deception," *Annals of Internal Medicine* 104 (1986):259-60.

37   For instance, medical journals make special efforts to avoid errors in drug dosages reported in journal articles by submitting them to additional proofreadings.

2

Misrepresentation of Data and the Integrity of Research

Paul J. Friedman

Misrepresentation is merely a polite word for lying. Lying about experimental results is a violation of the ethical code of a scientist. It contradicts the basic aim of scientific inquiry--to elucidate truth. It also violates the trust of colleagues, who expect a faithful reporting of results even if they do not believe the interpretation. False reporting may lead to improper or dangerous health-care decisions, as well as wasted money and effort on the part of those who try to make use of such results. Revelations of misrepresentation destroy the faith of the public in science and scientists. And, because science is so dependent for support on the good will and understanding of the public and its elected representatives, this is a disservice to the entire scientific enterprise. Finally, when making claims to a governmental agency, lying is against the law, and punishable by stiff penalties. It is no wonder that distinguished scientists as well as politicians have so firmly condemned misrepresentation and falsification.

Who would misrepresent data? It would have to be someone whose need for success or motivation for a specific outcome was overwhelming, or who was sufficiently out of touch with reality to risk personal reputation and that of science to achieve some personal goal. It would have to be someone with a weak moral sense, someone who failed to absorb (or chose to ignore) the norms of science in all his or her years of training. Distinguished scientists agree that such individuals--and fortunately there are few of them--have no place in science, and should be denounced and banished when their misdemeanors are discovered. Clearly, it is the responsibility of scientists at all levels to maintain the integrity of research by reporting any evidence of misrepresentation. In addition, it is generally agreed that the literature should be "cleansed" by retracting work that has been tainted by misrepresentation.

SECOND THOUGHTS

My goal here was to describe, without intentional exaggeration, the orthodox approach of science to the idea of misrepresentation of data. This straightforward approach runs into complications if the issues are analyzed more carefully.

For example, if one probes the mind of the perpetrator of untruths more closely, the question naturally arises, does he or she believe in his or her own misrepresentation? The orthodox answer would be, of course not. Is a liar fooled by his or her own lies? Yet this is an unsatisfactory answer, because human experience teaches us that individuals are often deceived by their own dreams or boasts. Scientific experience reveals that self-deception is a common source of laboratory error. Much of what we call the scientific method is an attempt to counter the biases that result from such self-deception. There also is a difference between false data and false conclusions, which affects the culpability of the responsible scientist. How can a reviewing authority determine whether an individual's false reporting of data is intentional or inadvertent? To judge responsibly, I believe it is necessary to judge intent, which is much more of a challenge than to judge only the facts. This issue is mentioned in Patricia Woolf's chapter, "Distinguishing Between Error and Fraud," which emphasized the importance of this difference, and in Jules Hallum's chapter, "Current Concerns of the Office of Scientific Integrity," in which he indicates that intent is outside the definition of scientific misconduct and beyond the scope of official evaluation by the Office of Scientific Integrity.

RECOGNIZING MISREPRESENTATION

Just as there are "black" lies and "white" lies, so there are fraud and lesser sins. A variety of colorfully named practices--fudging, cooking, trimming--describe alterations of data for more favorable presentation. Selection of data according to its perceived reliability is an integral part of experimental research, but is commonly a subjective exercise. It is usually difficult to determine after the fact whether unfavorable data were dropped in the interests of greater accuracy or to support the hypothesis (or both). Treatment of outliers in statistical analysis is not "cut and dried." In clinical research, some patient characteristics may be ignored to qualify them for a protocol, or may be kept in when their compliance is imperfect. Is it not a good idea to include a few extra animals or experiments so you can delete the worst results before running your statistics? What are the boundaries of good practice? When is selective reporting of data a result of misrepresentation, or of unconscious bias, or of critical laboratory work? Context also influences the definition or identification of misrepresentation. Although there is widespread agreement that it is irresponsible to misrepresent data in a published peer-reviewed paper (even more so because the reviewers evaluate the paper under the assumption that the author believes everything he has written), there is equally widespread cynicism about what appears in abstracts or proceedings of meetings. Many scientists go beyond their data when they prepare abstracts, but no one appears to regard this as culpable misrepresentation. There is a fine line between enthusiastic release of early results and premature reporting of conclusions; however, neither is without cost if more thorough research would have changed the outcome. Similarly, the reporting of "preliminary results" in research grant applications often is an exercise in favorable data selection, specifically intended to influence reviewers to provide funds for additional experiments. Is this misrepresentation? If this practice is wrong, then it is a dangerous thing to do; it is a federal crime to lie on a federal grant application. More subtle forms of misrepresentation can also be found in research grant applications. Scientists who think they are on the verge of something really promising will not put down what they really know and intend to do, for fear of being "scooped" by an unscrupulous competitor reviewing their application. Others use the traditional ploy of asking for money to do work that they essentially have completed, intending to use the grant award to support new work that is not described in the application. These are deliberate attempts to mislead grant reviewers for the federal granting agencies about data; that is, misrepresentation. Yet, these practices can hardly be called reprehensible; no responsible scientist would denounce someone for these customary practices.

MISREPRESENTATION FROM NATURE OR NURTURE: THE RESEARCH ENVIRONMENT

Are there individuals who have grown up deficient in ethical sense, and who are therefore untrainable? Are there more individuals now working in science than in the past with character disorders or serious personality disturbances? Probably there is no greater proportion of such individuals, but there are likely to be more in absolute number because of the growth of the scientific enterprise. Are these the persons who commit the rare but conspicuous acts of fraud or misrepresentation that have been publicized? Unfortunately, the "bad apple" argument has been used as an excuse for denying the existence of ethical problems in scientific research, and has therefore become discredited. Nevertheless, the most egregious frauds have shown symptoms of foolhardiness and self-destruction that are hard to reconcile with a normal personality structure. It has been argued that less serious but more common acts of misrepresentation have a greater deleterious effect on research.[1] Therefore, attempts to raise standards should focus on the great majority of scientists, especially those whose formal training in research is inadequate.

The willingness to bend the facts to serve goals other than the objective pursuit of truth is certainly a function of ethical and moral development. It has been argued that adults' ethical standards are as developed as they are going to be, and that training in ethics, for example, is unlikely to influence behavior. There is survey evidence that past courses or discussions about research ethics do not influence respondents' predictions of whether they might cheat in the future.[2] However, there is also evidence that the moral maturity of medical students measurably changes with training, and that some methods are more effective than others.[3] With increased attention to teaching ethics and more sophistication about how to do it, research scientists may develop greater sensitivity to the importance of observing strict standards of data handling and reporting.

How do ordinary scientists develop their ethical standards? It seems likely that young scientists learn their behavioral norms at the same time they learn the technical side of science. As they practice laboratory techniques, they also observe how the enterprise of science is pursued: what you have to do to obtain publications, research grants, faculty appointments, and tenure. They do not have to look far to see that not all scientists have equivalent ethical standards. Trainees are also keenly aware of the increasingly competitive environment. They recognize the importance of getting good research results to win federal support and the necessity of compromising traditional scientific openness to obtain commercial support or simply to avoid being beaten by the competition. Misrepresentation in some form may be a deliberate choice through a (mis?)perception of necessity or a combination of pressures. For example, trainees indicated greater likelihood of cheating to get research grants than in research publications.[4] Choices are not made in a vacuum; any decision will depend on an admixture of prior ethical standards, the prevailing scientific ethics of the local research environment, pressures for funding and advancement, the ethics of society outside the laboratory, and fear of the consequences of being discovered. It is the responsibility of scientific mentors and leaders to push this balance in the direction of higher ethical standards.

Research for industry and the resultant conflicts of interest affect the ethical tone of the environment. Although the ultimate benefit of much biomedical research depends on commercialization, the relatively recent idea that biological scientists could "strike it rich" in their laboratories has clearly altered the way scientists behave--for the worse. Scientific disputes, even accusations of misrepresentation, can occasionally be traced to an ambition to profit from discoveries. It is evident that some scientists can unlearn traditional high ethical standards. Careful institutional regulations and safeguards can help with conflict of interest, as is described in other chapters of this volume, but a balance is necessary to avoid overburdening creative individuals with excessive bureaucracy. Unfortunately, there is little that scientists can do about the degeneration of the ethical environment outside the laboratory, in both the increasingly business-oriented university and our morally deteriorating society.

MISREPRESENTATION ON THE GRAND SCALE

After hearing Professor Rustum Roy speak,[5] it is no longer possible to think of misrepresentation merely in the context of individual experiments or papers. He has forcefully shown how science has consistently misrepresented the potential of its discoveries to the public in order to secure continued generous support. The promise of high technology has been oversold, with the enthusiastic help of journalists, so that scientists learn to ignore most of the speculation that accompanies the announcement of each "breakthrough." The "big science" items are typically the worst; it is hard not to be embarrassed by the tales of miracles to be expected from the genome-mapping project,[6] or how we will finally be able to understand it all with the help of the superconducting super collider. In this environment, it is easier to understand how the individual scientist learns to exaggerate, to select, to misrepresent, in order to achieve the worthy goals of continued funding and growth.

RESPONDING TO SUSPICION OR EVIDENCE OF MISREPRESENTATION

Scientists are not eager to accuse colleagues of misrepresentation. Among colleagues, they are more likely to dismiss someone's work as wrong or misguided, and to openly criticize conclusions and data. In public, it is unusual to hear accusations that work has been misrepresented; however, in private, there are some laboratories and scientists whose work is sufficiently suspect that it is not trusted by those in the know. Some journals have blacklists of authors whose work is considered by the editor to be too untrustworthy to publish, but it is not publicly challenged as dishonest. Reporting such suspicions to the author's institution is uncommon. There is more than scientific caution in this reserve; there is also fear of lawsuits and the difficulty of proving misrepresentation, either before other scientists or before the law.

The same reservations affect the individual who might bring charges about work that is suspect. Suspicion is one thing; proof is another. Proof by scientific standards must be strong enough to overwhelm assumptions about lack of intent to misrepresent. On the other hand, the institutional official must not take into account the intent of the person bringing charges of misrepresentation; the evidence is what counts. Legitimate skepticism should result in dismissal of charges if the evidence does not eliminate the possibility that the misrepresentation was fortuitous or unintentional. This strong benefit of the doubt is not the standard of the law in civil cases, however. This is but one reason it is better to take care of misconduct cases within the research institution rather than in the courts--"preponderance of the evidence" is not good enough for scientific proof.

Are scientists denounced for "lesser sins" by their peers? As science becomes more self-conscious about research misconduct, there are more charges of improper behavior, but (with some important exceptions) these tend to come from junior scientists or laboratory personnel rather than true peers. Scientific colleagues seem to be highly tolerant of various degrees of misrepresentation. Perhaps working scientists take a more restrained view than their spokesmen because they are less confident about what constitutes deliberate and culpable misrepresentation. There are several attitudes that inhibit publicly demanding higher standards. Such views include "everybody does it," "it doesn't affect the results," concern about having to carry the burden of proof, fear of retribution, and a desire not to make trouble for a colleague. It is not the American way to tell tales. There is also caution about publicly acknowledging that all is not as advertised in science, that some scientists are not so dedicated to the truth as much as to priority, prestige, and power. Recommendations from within the academy that research ethics might need some attention[7] have received abundant criticism from others concerned about public reaction to this admission. There is a sensible reserve in not letting a few sensational revelations cripple the mighty machine of modern science. But events tend to escape this careful control. Can the public cope with the discovery that scientists are not saints? Let us hope so. Rather than try to repair the damage of misrepresentation by denial, science has to try to educate the public to its reality.

In summary, both ideal and customary responses depend on a graded perception of the seriousness of the misrepresentation and the costs of being critical or accusatory, as well as a sense of what the consequences will be for the accused. The seriousness of consequences for what many regard as minor transgressions surely inhibits accusations; unfortunately, many cases of serious misrepresentation have started with what appeared to be minor misdeeds. To catch these cases early requires more open criticism with less severe penalties for those whose errors, deliberate or indeterminate, are uncovered by these challenges.

NEW REGULATIONS, NEW PRESSURES

Although the scientific community is finally giving serious attention to the issue of misrepresentation, there is no consensus on whether a significant problem exists. The amount of attention is a result of external pressure on the scientific establishment and its granting agencies, originally brought by the press, then by muck-raking Congressmen and their reformist scientist assistants. More embarrassing than the publicized cases of misrepresentation was the difficulty that academic institutions had in dealing with them and with those accusers who brought abuses to public attention. Denial was the dominant psychological or administrative response for some years; indeed, we still indulge in denial whenever possible. For many years, the National Institutes of Health used benign neglect to treat this problem, until forced by Congressional pressure to take it seriously. One of the results was a set of regulations instructing grantee institutions on their responsibilities in responding to charges of misconduct;

another was the creation of the Office of Scientific Integrity, which Jules Hallum describes in his chapter and, with typical government overkill, simultaneous creation of an Office of Scientific Integrity Review to "look over their shoulders."

Protection of complainants or whistleblowers has been an important feature of various regulations. However much scientists admire these provisions in the context of denouncing government waste and corruption, there is less enthusiasm about the whistleblower in the academic research laboratory. At worst, some regard such protections as a way for an incompetent worker to avoid dismissal--simply by bringing charges. At best, cautioning the indignant accused faculty member about the protected status of the despised complainant is personally awkward, though quite necessary, especially since it must be done long before the charges are found valid or unsubstantiated.

Additional regulations were proposed to require institutions to deal more conscientiously with conflict of interest; these were so burdensome and restrictive that they were quickly sent back to the drawing board. This subject is covered in considerable detail by other authors in this volume (see chapters by Porter, Korn, Mishkin, Neaves, and Hansen). Finally, a potentially important step was taken by the National Institutes of Health, joining the Alcohol, Drug Abuse, and Mental Health Administration (ADAMHA) in requiring that there be some instruction in research ethics to trainees supported on their training grants. These agencies wisely let the individual programs determine the appropriate strategy for their own environments, which will encourage imaginative, practical and effective programs, and facilitate development of teaching materials. Eventually, the government intends to recommend specific requirements in ethics education. The potential practical problems of rigid recipes for scientific training are massive. Unfortunately, this provides no coverage for the large number of informally trained medical researchers.

Scientists always ask for support for more research on the subject, any subject. Actually, we know little formally about how ethical norms of science are absorbed. It will require exploration of the research environment by social and behavioral scientists to understand more rigorously how scientists develop. The development of research trainees requires a skilled interpretive study like that done for young surgeons by Bosk.[8] Modifications of existing measurement techniques (cited by Self[9]) will be necessary to determine the effectiveness of the interventions that will now be widely implemented.

Another legislative action that has begun to have an effect in this area is the broadening of the False Claims Act. Now the much-abused whistleblower has a chance to gain not only a decent hearing--which much of the regulatory activity of the last couple of years has sought--but may also profit financially from showing that there has been misrepresentation to the federal government. Of course, this threatens to bring a variety of unhappy or disgruntled former employees out to take advantage of the opportunity. This involves dealing with lawyers and going to court, which is not a comfortable situation for scientists and administrators. Furthermore, while the law's definition of misrepresentation is not clear yet, it is likely that it will not be the same as the standard of most scientists.

SUMMARY

A graded response to misconduct or misrepresentation is needed. In the words of the poet, "let the punishment fit the crime." There is an underlying recognition, however, that those competent to judge have an interest in minimizing the impact of that judgment on their institutions and on public perceptions of science. This is a serious conflict of interest, but it is best dealt with by disclosure and discussion, not by moving these problems into the adversarial environment of the courts or abandoning all initiative to a federal agency. If faculty can handle peer review for publication, research funding, and academic advancement with such a high level of integrity and effectiveness, they can manage misconduct problems.

Definitions have been troublesome, and proposals--this one included--have been based on armchair wisdom rather than scientific study and analysis. There is widespread misunderstanding of how science works, some of which has been fostered by us. We can do better than we have in recent years in education of both the public and of those who will carry the traditions of science forward.

NOTES

1   Institute of Medicine, National Academy of Sciences, "The Responsible Conduct of Research in the Health Sciences, Report of a Study," (Washington, DC: National Academy Press, 1989).
2   M. Kalichman and P.J. Friedman, "Perceptions of Research Trainees Concerning Research Ethics: A Pilot Study," submitted for publication, 1992.
3   D.J. Self, F.D. Wolinsky, and J.D. Baldwin, "The Effect of Teaching Medical Ethics on Medical Students' Moral Reasoning," *Academic Medicine* 64 (1989):755-59.
4   Kalichman and Friedman, "Perceptions of Research Trainees Concerning Research Ethics: A Pilot Study."
5   R. Roy, "Constructive and Destructive Scientific Error vs. Fraud in Science," paper presented at Scientific Integrity: Institutional and Individual Responsibilities, a conference held in March 1991 at the Center for Academic Ethics, Wayne State University, Detroit.
6   D.B. Paul, "Enthusiastic Claims" (book review), *Science* 252 (1991): 1423.
7   Institute of Medicine, "The Responsible Conduct of Research."
8   C. Bosk, *Forgive and Remember* (Chicago: University of Chicago Press, 1981).
9   Self, Wolinsky, and Baldwin, "The Effect of Teaching Medical Ethics."

3

Treatment of Allegations of Research Misconduct by American Universities

Allan Mazur

For years, a story about two paragons of physics, Nobel Prize-winning physicist Hans Bethe (pronounced "Beta") and famed mathematician George Gamow, circulated among scientists as an amusing piece of folklore. It seems that Gamow and another scientist named Alpher had written an article, which they sent to Bethe, asking that he join them in authorship. Bethe agreed, although he had made no contribution to the paper, so that the authorship line would read "Alpher, Bethe, Gamow." The story is true, as Bethe attested to me. I used to think that the significance of this anecdote lay in what it told us about the scientific sense of humor. Today I think it is more important as an example of behavior that was once regarded as wholly moral and worthy of applause, but if done today would be regarded by many as research misconduct, perhaps even as plagiarism.

Since 1980, there has been an unusual number of reports in the news media of misconduct in scientific research, especially the bedrock abuses of falsification of data and plagiarism. No one knows if these represent "the tip of the iceberg" or "a few bad apples," but in either case they represent a challenge to universities, medical schools, and other institutions that conduct or support research. Whereas in the past, if such incidents arose, they could be ignored or

This paper discusses research undertaken for, and funded by, the Project on Scientific Fraud and Misconduct of the American Association for the Advancement of Science and the American Bar Association, National Conference of Lawyers and Scientists. Results have been published previously in the project's "Report on Workshop Number Two" (Washington, DC: American Association for the Advancement of Science, 1989), and in A. Mazur, "Allegations of Dishonesty in Research and their Treatment by American Universities," *Minerva* 27 (Summer-Autumn 1989): 177-94.

handled privately and informally, this is no longer true. Their increased visibility today, the increased number of parties interested in these cases, and the threat of lawsuits have forced more openness and propriety in the treatment of allegations of misconduct. This has been a painful process; first, because of ambiguous and shifting notions of what constitutes misconduct; and second, because scientific institutions have not yet evolved methods of treatment that are generally accepted today.

A MODEL OF PROPRIETY

Recently, several universities, professional organizations, and federal governmental bodies have proposed explicit procedures for dealing with allegations of research misconduct.[1] These generally provide that the institutions should prepare a formal statement of policy that stipulates standards for honesty in research and procedures for dealing with allegations of misconduct, including a clear location of responsibility for investigation of alleged misconduct. They all stress that investigations should be prompt and that the proceeding should be recorded in detail if it appears that the allegations are not frivolous or obviously mistaken, and that a formal investigation should be undertaken by scientifically qualified individuals who are not close associates of the accused person. They provide too that the accused scientist should have a full opportunity to answer the allegations made against him, and that, furthermore, the allegations should remain confidential to protect the reputation of the person under suspicion until there is a reasonable certainty that misconduct has indeed occurred. Persons who first disclose the malpractice--"whistleblowers"--should be protected against reprisals unless their actions are frivolous. Then, if misconduct is established, all institutions outside the university that have been connected with the research or that might become connected with it, such as journals and funders, should be notified.

Some university and medical school administrators disagree with these proposed procedures,[2] and even among those who do agree there is uncertainty about how they should be implemented. Nonetheless, I have accepted these procedures as a model for properly handling an allegation of research misconduct, and in the remainder of this paper regard any serious departure from it as an instance of mishandling.

RESPONSES OF UNIVERSITIES

How have universities responded when confronted with allegations of fraud or misconduct on the part of members of their staffs? In some instances, the institutions have been severely criticized, sometimes for taking allegations too lightly and sometimes for violating the rights of people involved.

I will address here cases that have been made public. Several investigators, including Patricia Woolf, have compiled excellent lists of such instances, which are highly redundant, and I accept them as a reliable canvass of allegations that appear in the public literature.[3] I have selected from among these the cases where the alleged misconduct occurred at an American university, medical school, or institution with similar research traditions, with public disclosure after 1970 (but none later than 1987), and where there are reasonable grounds to believe that the allegation is at least partly correct. I include only cases where the accused held a doctorate or was a doctoral student. The result is 21 cases, which are the basis for my analysis.[4] Of these instances, 90 percent occurred in biomedical research, which is certainly much more than the percentage of all scientific research that is biomedical in nature. It is a plausible although untested contention that the norms and conditions of biomedical science foster more cheating than do those in other fields of research.[5] It is also possible that the apparently high incidence of biomedical misconduct is an artifact, and that biomedical misconduct is simply most likely to be reported and publicized in the news media. In any case, medical schools are the place in the university that is most involved in these cases and most criticized for inadequacies in the way allegations are treated.

For most of these cases of research misconduct, I have no reason to suspect mishandling by the university of the allegations, simply because I have too little information on the procedures that were followed. It is certainly possible that major improprieties occurred but escaped public attention. In only a minority of cases is there sufficient public information to make a reasonable judgement about whether or not allegations were handled properly.

The case of the radiologist, Robert Slutsky, who was accused of falsification of data at the medical school of the University of California at San Diego, is an instance of the proper handling of allegations.[6] While Slutsky's publications were being reviewed in preparation for a decision on his academic promotion, a senior member of the radiology department noticed apparent discrepancies in different reports on the same laboratory animals. Asked to account for these discrepancies, Slutsky responded that he could not locate his original data. He then resigned from the university.

Following the rules established after earlier cases of misconduct, the university promptly created an investigative committee that found that, in at least three papers, data had been fabricated. A second committee was formed to examine a complete set of Slutsky's publications, which he had been producing at a rate of about one paper every 10 days. Of these, 10 additional papers were deemed fraudulent and 53 others were called of "questionable validity."

Although the press had been informed by unknown persons of the investigation at an early stage, reporters agreed to await definitive conclusions before announcing the scandal. The university sent notification of the fraudulent and questionable papers to all relevant scientific journals, funding bodies, and coauthors. Slutsky was offered an opportunity to retract these, and he did eventually withdraw 15 published papers, but he did not acknowledge that he had committed fraud.

Not all allegations are treated with this care. According to public testimony by credible individuals, 8 of the 21 cases known to me were incorrectly dealt with by the institution in which the fraud was allegedly perpetrated. These cases of mishandling, described in detail elsewhere,[7] fit three patterns; I will describe these patterns, along with an exemplar for each type.

THREE PATTERNS OF MISHANDLING

In one pattern, which I call "old boy damage control," the dishonesty is allegedly committed by a relatively junior person in the laboratory of a prestigious senior scientist, and the two have a close relationship, perhaps as protege and mentor. The initial response of the senior scientist is disbelief; then an attempt is made to prevent a public scandal by dealing with the case quietly within a narrow circle of immediate associates or other senior people--the "old boys." In these cases, the senior scientists--at least initially--take it upon themselves to assess the allegations, despite their own close connection with the persons and work in question, and this may cloud their judgments, leading them to minimize the degree of misconduct. In each instance of this kind, the involvement of outsiders forces an enlargement of the inquiry, to the subsequent embarrassment of the senior scientists and their institutions. The well-known case of John Darsee is an exemplar.

Darsee was a rapidly rising protege and frequent coauthor of Professor Eugene Braunwald, an eminent cardiologist who was physician in chief of two of the most prominent hospitals associated with Harvard Medical School. Some other young scientists in Braunwald's laboratory were dubious about Darsee's huge list of publications and, in 1981, after witnessing him fabricate data, they brought their case against him to Dr. Robert Kloner, who acted as director of the laboratory during Braunwald's absences. Darsee admitted the fabrication of these data, but insisted that his other work had been honest. In response, Professor Braunwald withdrew his proposal that Darsee be appointed to the Harvard faculty, but he allowed Darsee to continue work--now under closer supervision--on a multi-laboratory study supported by the National Institutes of Health (NIH), and to continue to submit his papers for publication. No external organization, even the NIH, was notified of the incident.

Over the next four months, Braunwald and Kloner examined Darsee's other work in their laboratory and concluded that it was accurate. Meanwhile, scientists at the NIH noticed that data collected by Darsee for his part of the multi-laboratory study diverged from the results obtained by workers at the other laboratories. Dr. Kloner noticed this discrepancy at about the same time, and only then did he notify NIH that Darsee had earlier been observed in dishonest conduct.

Harvard Medical School and NIH appointed panels of inquiry. The report of the Harvard panel is widely regarded as a whitewash, exonerating Darsee and justifying the actions of Braunwald and Kloner. The NIH report was critical of Harvard's handling of the case, including Braunwald and Kloner's failure to recognize anomalies in Darsee's other work in their laboratory, and their permitting him to continue work on the multi-laboratory project without notifying NIH that he had cheated on a project which it supported. Professor Braunwald has maintained a vigorous defense of his own behavior.

In a second pattern of mishandling, which I call "the abrasive whistle-blower," the allegation is made by someone who is relatively junior, or at least less senior than the alleged wrongdoer. Apparently, the charges are raised in a way that appears petty or vindictive to the person hearing them, leading to a suspicion that the whistleblower is motivated by jealousy or personal animosity. As a result, the allegations are discounted and, in some cases, even boomerang into threats against the whistleblower, especially if the accused is well thought of by those hearing the charges. Often the alleged misconduct is confirmed only because of the persistence of these whistleblowers, who may bring in the news media to coerce inhospitable authorities to pursue the allegations.

One such whistleblower is Bruce Hollis, who in 1980, while a post-doctoral fellow in endocrinology at Case Western Reserve University, became suspicious of research by his immediate superior, Dr. Philip Lambert. Hollis expressed his concerns to higher authorities in the institution; he thought that nearly everyone ignored his statements and was displeased with him for making them. By 1982, after leaving Dr. Lambert's laboratory for another position at the university, Hollis became concerned over the fact that Lambert was including his name on publications reporting research upon which he, Hollis, had never worked. At a national meeting, Hollis let it be known that he could not attest to the results reported in papers to which his name had been attached. In response, Dr. Lambert insisted on an investigation to clear his name, while superiors at the university warned Hollis against continuing his attack on Lambert.

An inquiry initiated by the university, which was later criticized by the NIH for lacking in both timeliness and quality, blamed both Lambert and Hollis for inept research practices in Lambert's laboratory. Hollis says he was not given a full opportunity to defend himself during the investigation, and that the investigating committee failed to consult individuals who could--and later did--resolve conflicting testimony. Hollis received notice that his academic appointment would be terminated.

Until 1984, the NIH had not been involved, but--once the case was reported in the *Cleveland Plain Dealer*--it then began its own investigation, with the result that Hollis was cleared of wrongdoing while future financial support for Lambert was restricted. In response, the university reappointed Hollis, but he soon resigned and took an appointment elsewhere.

I call the third pattern of institutional mishandling "dilution of responsibility." Here the alleged misconduct does not occur within the boundaries of a single institution that has the authority and responsibility to investigate it. As a result, no one takes the initiative to conduct a full inquiry, so investigations are incomplete, slovenly, and either perfunctory or excessively prolonged. The case of Elias Alsabti is a remarkable example where no institution was concerned about misconduct outside its own walls.

Alsabti, a young and wealthy Middle Easterner claiming relationship to the Jordanian royal family, came to the United States in 1977 to complete his medical training and pursue a career as a researcher. He moved to Temple University, claiming to have a successful but secret vaccine for leukemia. When his incompetence became clear, he was asked to leave, so he moved to Jefferson Medical College, also in Philadelphia, working in the lab of microbiologist Frederick Wheelock, who was unaware of the problems at Temple. Soon, evidence that Alsabti was making up data became so strong that he was asked to leave Jefferson too. Again, the affair was kept quiet. In leaving, Alsabti took some of Wheelock's manuscripts and later published sections of them as his own.

Alsabti moved next to M.D. Anderson Hospital in Houston. By now, he was frequently publishing--or republishing--in journals around the world, simply retyping someone else's already published paper, listing himself as author, and sending the piece out to an obscure journal. In one instance, Alsabti obtained a preliminary manuscript from someone, sent it out to a Japanese journal with a new title under his own authorship, and had it published before the original author did.

When one instance of plagiarism was proved at M.D. Anderson, Alsabti was asked to leave there too. He moved to Houston's South West Memorial Hospital, having supplied excellent references. In the meantime, he completed work for an MD degree "in absentia" from the American University of the Caribbean. In 1980, he was accepted into a medical residency at the University of Virginia.

By this time, some of the plagiarized authors had become aware that their research had been stolen. Wheelock wrote to Alsabti about the work that had been plagiarized from Jefferson Medical College. Alsabti responded that Wheelock was insulting his integrity and threatened legal action. Wheelock then wrote a letter to four major journals, explaining the plagiarism, but only the *Lancet* published his notice; most editors regarded the instance as a personal affair between Wheelock and Alsabti. By then, the snowball of concern had grown to a size that warranted exposé articles about Alsabti in *Science* and *Nature* and then elsewhere. Alsabti responded with countercharges that other researchers had pirated his papers. He also objected to the inaccuracy of the

Science piece, which claimed that he had a yellow Cadillac, when in fact it was white! By then, mid-1980, Alsabti was working on a residency at a hospital affiliated with Boston University, but when officials there read the news, he was again asked to leave. This time, he apparently left the country, perhaps to continue his career back in the Middle East.

WHAT CAN BE DONE?

We are now in an awkward period, when traditional practices of universities and medical schools in treating alleged misconduct are inadequate, and satisfactory new practices have not yet evolved. There are successful instances--such as the way in which the University of California at San Diego handled the Slutsky case--but these have not yet become the norm. Scientists and administrators, presented with allegations of misconduct, are grasping for the proper means to conduct themselves. I am afraid that in their uncertainty, and to protect themselves from both embarrassment and lawsuits, some have moved too quickly to convert academic inquiries, the province of scientists and professors, into legal inquiries directed by lawyers. I have followed closely one recent case concerning academic misconduct of a relatively minor kind, where the early entry of lawyers for both sides produced a polarization and escalation that have made the incident far more costly for everyone than it need have been.

Observed patterns of mishandling suggest solutions that can be implemented by universities without relinquishing control to lawyers. Clearly, senior scientists ought to remove themselves from investigations of alleged misconduct within their own laboratories. This is a lot to ask of a powerful lab chief, especially in the early stages of a potential scandal that could blemish the reputation of the lab and its leadership, but this must become a standard of behavior in such situations. It is natural that people in positions of authority discount accusations made in an offensive manner by people of low standing. Although the personal manner and motives of the accuser are not the criteria by which to assess the truth or falsity of accusations, it is difficult to hold them separate. Accusations ought to be made in a temperate and matter-of-fact way.

No matter how much improvement can be made in the universities' treatment of alleged misconduct, we may all agree that the best solution is to minimize the occurrence of misconduct in the first place. No one knows the frequency with which scientific investigators behave dishonestly, and there have been several proposals to determine that frequency, perhaps by an audit of published research reports. Such efforts are unlikely to be very successful because of the uncertain boundary between acceptable and unacceptable practices, as in the Alpher-Bethe-Gamow authorship, and because many forms of falsification are practically undetectable. Even if one could establish the amount of improper behavior, it would not make much difference for science policy, unless that amount were implausibly high. More importantly, establishing the frequency of misconduct in research would not tell us why it occurs or how to cure it.

It would be more fruitful (and more feasible) to investigate the relative occurrence of dishonesty in different branches of science, especially in biomedical research as compared to other areas of work. Results of such studies would indicate if the primary causes of dishonesty are widespread in our scientific institutions, or are concentrated in a subset of them, which operate differently from the others. These results would be useful in formulating a strategy to deal with fraud in research, telling us whether to concentrate efforts on the special conditions that have developed in the biomedical research institutions, or to deal more broadly with the general activity of research.

NOTES

1   Mazur, "Allegations of Dishonesty in Research," 179.
2   P. Greene, J. Durch, W. Horwitz, and V. Hooper, "Policies for Responding to Allegations of Fraud in Research," *Minerva* 23 (Summer 1985):203-15.
3   W. Broad and N. Wade, *Betrayers of the Truth* (New York: Simon and Schuster, 1982); A. Kohn, *False Prophets* (New York: Basil Blackwell, 1986); P. Woolf, "Deception in Scientific Research," *Jurimetrics* 29 (Fall 1988):67-95.
4   Mazur, "Allegations of Dishonesty in Research."
5   J. Swazey and S. Sher, *Whistleblowing in Biomedical Research* (Washington, DC: US Government Printing Office, 1981).
6   E. Marshall, "San Diego's Tough Stand on Research Fraud," *Science* 234 (1986):534; P. Friedman, "Fraud in Radiological Research," *American Journal of Radiology* 150 (January 1988):27.
7   Mazur, "Allegations of Dishonesty in Research."

4

Office of Scientific Integrity: Why, What, and How

Jules V. Hallum and Suzanne W. Hadley

Recently, comments have been made concerning the perceived "Big Brother" control over science by the Office of Scientific Integrity (OSI). The purpose of this chapter is to describe why the OSI was formed, what it is, how it functions, and what philosophy guides its actions. In this way, the scientific community can judge for itself the purpose and methods of the OSI and decide on the basis of fact, rather than hearsay, whether the OSI should be an active participant in the scientific dialogue.

The establishment of the OSI in the Office of the Director of the National Institutes of Health (NIH) was announced in the Federal Register.[1] Its responsibilities, as well as the responsibilities of awardee and applicant institutions for dealing with and reporting possible misconduct in science, were described in the so-called Final Rule.[2]

The forces that converged to cause these actions were social, political, and professional in origin. Social reaction to the more notorious and well-publicized cases of misconduct was seen to be eroding public confidence in science. Political concern for the public's loss of confidence in science was viewed by the Congress as potentially weakening the American scientific effort. Professional societies, such as the American Society for Microbiology, the Association of American Medical Colleges, and the American Association for the Advancement of Science, had a long-standing concern about scientific misconduct, not only because of its erosive effect on public support, but also because of its divisive effect on trust among scientists.

This chapter has been reproduced from an article that first appeared in *American Society for Microbiology News* 56, no.12 (1990):647-51. It is based on a presentation by Suzanne Hadley at the 1990 American Society for Microbiology Annual Meeting.

FINAL RULE

It was in response to these forces that the Final Rule was promulgated. The Final Rule contains several significant elements, three of which are of major importance to the present discussion.

The rule defines scientific misconduct as "fabrication, falsification, plagiarism, or other practices that seriously deviated from those that are commonly accepted within the scientific community for proposing, conducting, or reporting research." Specifically, misconduct does not include honest error or honest differences in interpretations or judgments of data. The rule establishes the OSI and the Office of Scientific Integrity Review (OSIR) as two independent but complementary elements of the Public Health Service's (PHS) effort for dealing with alleged and confirmed cases of scientific misconduct.

The rule requires that any institution applying for, or receiving, PHS funds for research have in place policies and procedures developed by the institution itself, to deal with allegations or suspected scientific misconduct. Institutions are required to submit an annual assurance to the OSI about their compliance with this aspect of the Final Rule.

The scientific community has been concerned about the loss of public trust over the past few years. The Three Mile Island and Chernolbyl debacles raised questions about the safety of these plants, which should, in the public's opinion, have been anticipated by scientists. The perceived role of science in the industrial pollution that threatens our entire planet and the idea that scientists are inhumane to animals also have contributed to this loss of respect.

That this is unfair to science is almost irrelevant. As scientists, we are perceived to be irresponsible and uncaring. Clearly, our responsibility as citizen-scientists in these matters was a significant one and one that we failed to meet. We did not accomplish what, in retrospect, should have been a duty for us. We have not done a good job of educating our fellow citizens or even ourselves on the ethical responsibilities we bring to our work. Surely, this must be a major challenge for the immediate future of science. Restoring the public trust in science is also a clear matter of self-interest, since eventually our purse strings are held by the public. Restoring this trust is a serious issue for all scientists.

Most of us believe that acts of scientific misconduct are rare instances. But is this really true? Even if it is, a single notorious case can have dramatic and costly impact on public perceptions of science, as seen in recent years. The OSI is dealing with approximately 80 active cases of alleged misconduct. In the 18 months since its creation, the OSI has resolved about 75 cases. While we do not know precisely the "denominator" for these figures, it is reasonable to assume that the public believes the fraction of dishonest scientists is significant and presents a very serious problem.

THE IMPORTANCE OF PUBLIC PERCEPTIONS

The new PHS regulations embodied in the Final Rule can be interpreted as an attempt to do something about the public perception of science and scientists as irresponsible careerists. Too, science is a multibillion-dollar enterprise with a major impact on the health and lifestyles of all of us, and on the state of the biosphere. We perhaps should not be surprised that an enterprise of this magnitude and impact became subject to regulation, as has occurred with other important enterprises. Given that these regulations are now fact, the question becomes, how can the regulations be managed to prevent them from inhibiting the creative aspects of science? Put another way, can science govern itself? We in the OSI believe that the answer clearly is "yes."

We all remember the serious debate that occurred when the provisions of the Final Rule were first discussed two years ago. The scientific community showed a pronounced resistance to any controls on science from any sector that was not itself a part of that community. It was largely in response to this concern that the OSI was established within NIH in a manner similar to that of the Office for Protection from Research Risks and the Office of Recombinant DNA Technology. Both of these offices have succeeded in their missions because they are part of the scientific community; as such, they include an emphasis on the review of scientific issues in their decisions. In a similar fashion, the professional staff of the OSI are all trained scientists who bring their training to bear on the scientific dialogue as it pertains to issues of possible misconduct.

Have the new policies and procedures for dealing with misconduct had any effect on the frequency of its occurrence? It is much too soon to attempt to answer that question. Logically, one might assume they have, if only by bringing the concern of the institutions for the responsible conduct of research to the attention of their constituencies. But more importantly, the existence of these policies and procedures could be expected to help solve a real problem.

When charges of scientific misconduct first became public knowledge a few years ago, many scientists were appalled at the poor quality of the misconduct investigations. To a significant extent, the lack of policy meant that investigating committees typically had little idea of what was expected of them. Too, the lack of established procedures led to inconsistencies, a lack of protection for "whistleblowers," and needless damage to the reputations of respondents (the accused). The new policies and procedures should encourage institutions to conduct better, fairer investigations. However, the question of whether institutions have the will to use these policies and procedures remains to be seen. A "sanitized" case from OSI files may serve as an example of that concern.

Dr. X went to a new job at B University after a postdoctoral experience with Professor Y at C University. A few years after this move, X wrote a paper on the work he had done with Y, without consulting Y or listing him as an author. Y read the paper and realized that some of the data presented were fabricated. Y wrote to B University and complained that the paper contained fabricated and falsified data. The university appointed a committee to consider the allegation. The committee neither looked at X's data books nor interviewed Dr. Y. They merely asked X to explain the allegations and wrote to the dean exonerating X. Y was not allowed to see the committee report. Dr. Y was persistent, however, and finally brought the case to the OSI, where a new investigation was undertaken. After extensive interviews of the complainant, respondent, and witnesses; examinations of data books by experts in the area of research under question; and study of all of the scientific facts involved, the OSI investigation showed clearly that there was serious misconduct on the part of Dr. X. The point of this example is that B University did not do a thorough and fair examination of the charges, largely, one supposes, because of a lack of will to investigate one of its own faculty.

THE ROLE OF THE NEW OSI

The OSI is best described by its responsibilities. It was established within NIH but has PHS-wide authority (including the Centers for Disease Control; Food and Drug Administration; Health Resources and Services Administration; Alcohol, Drug Abuse, and Mental Health Administration; and NIH) for both intra- and extramural research. The OSI has four major duties. The OSI:

1. Oversees implementation of all policies and procedures related to matters of possible scientific misconduct.
2. Oversees each investigation into alleged or suspected scientific misconduct conducted by any institution applying for, or receiving, PHS research funds.
3. Conducts inquiries or investigations when necessary.
4. Participates in and directs preventive and educational measures to encourage the responsible conduct of research. (As examples of this activity: the OSI has recently conducted a workshop for biomedical journal editors to determine ways in which the editors can interact with the OSI in matters related to suspected misconduct in scientific publications. In addition, a series of regional meetings are to be held this spring with institutional representatives to determine the institutions' experience during the first year of implementation of the Final Rule.)

How does the OSI work in cases of alleged scientific misconduct? Institutions are required to notify the OSI when, after an initial inquiry or fact-finding phase, a formal investigation will be undertaken. The OSI monitors the investigation for thoroughness, fairness, objectivity, and timeliness. Upon conclusion of the investigation, the OSI receives a full report on the institution's investigations citing the evidence, findings, conclusions, and sanctions imposed, if any. The OSI reviews the report and decides whether the findings of the investigation are fair and consistent with the evidence. If misconduct is confirmed and the OSI agrees, the report is forwarded, together with any additional sanctions imposed by the OSI, to the appropriate agency director, who then sends it to the OSIR for review. If the OSIR approves, it sends the report to the assistant secretary for health (ASH) for further review and a decision.

If the OSI does not accept the findings of an institution's investigation, it can ask that the institution reopen the investigation or can open its own inquiry or investigation.

The OSI can also open an inquiry or investigation following allegations made directly to the office. If an inquiry shows no evidence to warrant a formal investigation, the case can be closed at that time. If the inquiry demonstrates that there are facts to support an allegation that misconduct occurred, a formal investigation is initiated. The investigation is not simply an extended inquiry, but it is a formal process to determine whether scientific misconduct did occur, and if so, how serious it was and who was responsible. The same process is used both within PHS and for allegations of scientific misconduct in extramural research.

In both inquiries and investigations, the OSI is specifically charged with protecting the rights of the complainant and the reputation of the respondent. It does this in two ways. First, all of the deliberations and reports of the OSI are kept in the strictest confidence. Only when a finding of misconduct is proved and sanctions are approved by the ASH does the final report become available to the public.

If the respondent is found not to have committed an act of misconduct, the OSI offers a choice. The final report can be kept confidential, secure from release under the Freedom of Information Act; or, if the respondent wishes, perhaps because of media publicity, the OSI will work to help clear the respondent's reputation.

We previously asked the question of whether institutions will respect their policies and procedures regarding scientific misconduct. Another example, again properly fictionalized, will demonstrate the basis for the OSI's belief that institutions must share in this responsibility if science is to effectively govern itself.

At a major research university, a professor whose salary was 50 percent supported by PHS funds was charged with, and eventually admitted to, plagiarism. The university refused to provide its report on this matter to the OSI. The expressed reason was, in essence, that the scientist cheated on the non-PHS 50 percent of his time. Clearly, there is a serious question as to whether this university is following its own policies on scientific misconduct, and there is reason to believe the university is going to some lengths to protect a confessed plagiarist from sanctions by PHS.

The concern of the OSI is not simply for the particular case we have just described, but also for the question it raises: namely, if science refuses to govern itself, who will do the job? Both the Office of the Inspector General and the Department of Justice have been suggested. In Congress, a bill is being prepared that will make it necessary to have a courtlike process to investigate allegations of scientific misconduct.

TWO MODELS FOR DEALING WITH ALLEGED MISCONDUCT

Thus, after many months of dealing with instances of alleged scientific misconduct, two models of dealing with these cases seem to be emerging and competing. The first model to emerge might be termed the *scientific dialogue model*; this model has been used by the OSI in resolving all of its cases of possible scientific misconduct in its first 18 months of operation. The second model might be called the *legal adversary model*; it is the model espoused by many in the legal profession.

Both of these models have garnered sincere advocates. Both offer due process for those accused of misconduct; both provide protection of the American scientific enterprise. But each offers a different balance between these two elements--protection of science and due process protection of individuals--and thus have different advantages and disadvantages.

The legal adversary model clearly offers the most visible and obvious due-process protections. In this courtlike process, with its origins in Anglo-Saxon jurisprudence, the accused receives specific "charges" in writing, can be represented by counsel, can face and cross-examine all witnesses, and can introduce evidence on his or her own behalf. However, the role of scientists in such proceedings is likely to be minimized to that of "expert witnesses." This would represent a serious loss to the interests of science, because the issues are resolved on the basis of civil law or administrative law and not principally on scientific evidence. In addition, little protection of the anonymity of the whistleblower or reputation of the respondent is provided.

In dealing with issues of possible misconduct, the scientific dialogue model functions in much the same spirit as does an editor of a scientific journal in dealing with problems in a submitted manuscript. Theoretically, if any author makes a claim unsubstantiated by presentation of data, the editor can demand that those data be adduced or the paper will not be published. It is obvious to scientists, though perhaps not to laymen, that in this scientific dialogue the burden of proof must always fall on the person who makes claims about his or her data. If the data are provided, the other challenge is met; if not, the claim is not accepted by other scientists. The process is one of professional challenge to examine and evaluate data rather than an accusation per se. The OSI has followed this principle as its guiding philosophy since its inception in dealing with possible scientific misconduct. A scientist who is accused of misconduct is always asked to provide the data supporting the scientific findings that are at issue. This does not mean that the accused must bear the burden of proof to show that there is no misconduct. The absence of supporting data would not, alone, support a finding of misconduct. Such a finding by the OSI must be supported by evidence gathered during a thorough investigation of all pertinent scientific issues.

The scientific dialogue model, as implemented by the OSI, does indeed provide due process protections for those accused of misconduct. The respondent is notified by a confidential letter that an inquiry is bring made; and the scientific issues that are the focus of the inquiry are identified in the letter. As stated previously, the inquiry is a fact-finding effort, designed to determine whether evidence suggesting misconduct exists. If no such evidence is found, the inquiry is terminated and all parties concerned are notified, again, in confidence.

If, on the other hand, the inquiry results in a finding that an investigation is warranted, the respondent is notified, including specification of the issues identified by the OSI, and the process moves into a formal investigation phase.

In either an inquiry or investigation, all persons interviewed can be accompanied by counsel. The respondent can introduce evidence at any time and suggest witnesses to pertinent events. If the OSI uses a panel of expert scientific advisors in the investigation, as is common, the respondent can suggest scientists to serve on that panel. All pertinent witnesses as well as the respondent are interviewed, and the interviews are recorded. A full transcript of each interview is sent to the interviewee for correction, addition of comments, introduction of evidence or other material, and for refutation or rebuttal of previous evidence. This corrected transcript is used in the identification of issues and later in developing the findings of the investigation.

We believe it is evident that the scientific dialogue model does provide due-process protection. There is a significant difference from the legal adversary model. It is partly true that the OSI does not permit a direct confrontation or cross-examination of witnesses. The OSI is required by its regulations to maintain the highest degree of confidentiality to protect the whistleblower as well as the reputation of the respondent. However, the OSI does allow a full and open confrontation of scientific issues. The issues are identified and presented by the OSI in the course of its inquiry or investigation. The case belongs to the OSI at that time, not to the whistleblower. The issues as stated by the OSI are often different from, or more complex than, those brought in the original allegation. Thus, the OSI becomes a scientific arbiter, responsible for identifying and framing the issues. The OSI depersonalizes and institutionalizes the handling of the case. It is the issues of science identified by the OSI that must be responded to and resolved. The respondent meets with the OSI and is given the opportunity to rebut directly any evidence presented, with the advice of counsel, if desired. Thus, there is a direct confrontation, but of scientific issues, not individuals.

In the event that the results of an investigation point to misconduct, further due-process rights are provided. When a draft report of the findings is prepared, a copy is sent to the respondent for correction, comment, or rebuttal of evidence. This response must be considered and may lead to substantial charges in the report. In any event, it is appended to the final report.

If misconduct is confirmed and sanctions recommended, the respondent is informed of the proposed sanctions and afforded an opportunity to review and comment on them. The report is then subjected to review at three different levels, for thoroughness, fairness, and objectivity. The agency director, the OSIR, and the ASH all are responsible for ensuring that these criteria are met.

If, after all of these reviews, there is a recommendation for debarment (for a fixed time), an additional right, a formal hearing, is available to the respondent under Department of Health and Human Services regulation. The case is examined *de novo*, and the process then follows the legal adversary model, with an administrative judge provided and cross-examination of all witnesses allowed.

However, there is no comparable process beyond the three levels of review for lesser sanctions than debarment, since these sanctions (such as prevention from serving on an agency advisory panel, letter of reprimand, supervision of research, or certification of manuscripts and grants, all for a fixed time) are considered to be discretionary authorities of PHS agencies.

It is apparent that both of these models have special advantages and disadvantages. To some extent, the scientific community will help to decide which model should predominate. It is our opinion that if the adversary model, with its dependence on lawyers and legal rather than scientific determinations, should prevail, much will be lost. We believe that use of scientific dialogue in dealing with the occasional instances of possible scientific misconduct will best serve the public interest and the interest of science.

The OSI can function as part of the scientific dialogue only insofar as it is involved in this dialogue. This partnership involves participation at many levels. Scientists must be willing, when asked, to serve on the OSI advisory panels to help determine the issues of science involved in a case. Those who have served in this capacity to date have found it a challenging and interesting duty to science, and have expressed an admiration for the scientific fairness of the process.

Scientists must also recognize that they share responsibility for protecting PHS research funds. Universities must share in this responsibility, in their position as the leading producers of scientific research and researchers. The responsibility of institutions to inculcate students in responsible research practices is particularly crucial.

If partnership among the scientific community, the institutes and universities, and the OSI is properly ordered and maintained, it will provide a demonstration that science can indeed govern itself and thus help us to reestablish the high regard of science by the public and its representatives. The OSI is committed to this partnership.

NOTES

1   *Federal Register,* 16 March 1989, 11080.
2   *Federal Register,* 8 August 1989, 32446.

5

Authorship and Illustrations: The Challenge of Computer Manipulation

Paul J. Anderson

Scientific investigators who depend on documentary recording of morphological observations have relied on the traditional techniques of line art, photography, half-tone reproduction, and color separation for their publications. In such investigations (anatomy, histology, cell biology, hematology, and immunocytochemistry, to mention but a few) the illustrations are the data.

Probably every editor who works in morphology-dependent sciences has had to deal with the fraudulent use of illustrations, especially photographs.

A typical offense, for example, is to relabel a photograph from an earlier research project or publication and submit it as supporting data for a later manuscript. Common disguises include cropping, enlarging, reducing, and reversing or rotating the original image. Detection, though imperfect, is aided by study of an author's prior publications (for which manuscript referees are invaluable) and the fact that, like experiment data books, the author should have the original photographic negative in his or her possession.

The "original" negative, however, is rapidly being replaced by another kind of imaging data. The optical and chemical processes that have physically defined photography for a century and a half can now be ignored by using mathematically synthesized images on a computer.

The assumption that the recorded image is nature's mirror ("the camera does not lie") is being challenged by dramatic changes in image-making technology.[1] Videographic printouts, for example, closely resemble those produced by conventional film emulsions. Computer-stored images are easily manipulated to add or subtract details, modify colors, or combine subject matter from several sources. Image-generation formulas can now create computer images of a quality that appear to document "reality." Documentary support of scientific observation can thereby be customized. The printing industry increasingly uses computer scanners to prepare half tones that are easily adjusted to "improve" photographic copy to meet the demands of authors (and editors and publishers) who want "more contrast," "sharper lines," and "better resolution" of specific details. Production of color separations by laser scanning almost always "corrects" distortions in hue and color saturation in the original copy (usually in response to the perceived needs of authors, editors, and publishers). The problem is that such computer adjustments of illustrated copy are undocumented and undetectable.

Computer-assisted manipulation can occur at any stage of the publication process, from the creation of the original image by the author, through editorial adjustment of the illustration, to computer scanning of half tones and color separations during production. The wider availability and use of computer manipulation will inevitably raise the temptation to enhance illustrations for publication, so that they support investigative conclusions. This is especially true since such manipulation is virtually undetectable.[2]

Fred Ritchin, director of the photojournalism and documentary photography program of the International Center of Photography in New York, has stated the problem thus: "The computer is increasingly being used to manipulate the elements . . . and quickly and seamlessly rearrange them."[3]

I have no solutions for the problems involving the potential misuse of graphics' technology in scientific publication, but I would like to suggest several areas for immediate consideration.

As a first step, we should increase the awareness of the risks of computerized pictorial alteration among authors, editors, publishers, printers, and readers.

As it becomes easier to tamper with graphic evidence, all those involved in the process of publishing will have to vouch for the authenticity of the published image. Author, photographer, graphic artist, editor, publisher, and printer should be prepared to document the details of image production used in support of research conclusions.

Finally, those organizations concerned with publication standards should address the need for guidelines in the use of computer generated or manipulated graphics. Sanctions against the unethical use of illustrated materials produced by conventional techniques have been endorsed by several organizations (Graphic Artists' Guild,[4] Institute of Incorporated Photographers,[5] Council of Biology Editors[6]). Guidelines that confront the potential misuse of computer imaging in scientific documentation have yet to be developed.

NOTES

1   "New Picture Technologies Push Seeing Still Further from Believing," *New York Times*, 3 July 1989, p. 42.

2   F. Ritchin, "Photojournalism in the Age of Computers," in *The Critical Image*, ed. C. Squires (Seattle, WA: Bay Press, 1990), 28-37.

3   F. Ritchin, *In Our Own Image: The Coming Revolution in Photographs* (New York: Aperture Foundation, 1990).

4   Graphic Artists Guild, "Pricing and Ethical Guidelines," in *Graphic Arts Guild Handbook*, 7th ed. (New York: Graphic Artists Guild, 1991).

5   Institute of Incorporated Photographers, *Code of Professional Conduct* (Ware, MA: Institute of Incorporated Photographers, 1969).

6   Scientific Illustration Committee, "Legal and Ethical Considerations," in *Illustrating Science: Standards for Publication*, Chapter 11. (Bethesda, MD: Council of Biology Editors, 1988), 251-63.

6

Credit and Responsibility in Scientific Authorship

Addeane S. Caelleigh

Whose name appears on a scholarly paper's byline? The question of authorship is by no means a simple one, nor is it free of emotion and dispute. International committees meet and issue statements, conference panelists debate, and authors struggle among themselves and with editors about authorship. Those involved know that the stakes are high and that the answer involves serious issues.

Authorship looms large in discussions of scientific publishing because it focuses attention on the tension between the demands to receive due recognition for effort and the need to accept responsibility for the work. The issue concerns editors and authors because it can raise difficult ethical choices; it is of interest to the public because of the potential social consequences of such choices; and it is of general concern to a research community that must feel confident that what is said is accurate and that who says it is believable. As editors and authors and members of a community based on trust, we must remind ourselves of the need to focus on how credit for work should be rightly determined when selecting the authors for published science, and on how authors must take responsibility for the validity and truthfulness of published work.

CONTEXT

No one needs another exposition on the pressure to publish that science and university researchers feel. Most feel obliged to publish often and at length in approved journals if they wish to prosper in position and esteem. In science especially, the journal article is the customary measure in considering someone for a grant proposal, society membership, or academic promotion; articles and grants are the currency of a career. While we never merely weigh the bulk of accumulated articles in assigning virtue, it is clear that weight, as well as weightiness, are key elements in approval and reward.

There are eloquent descriptions of the pressure to publish and sound condemnations of its undesirable fruits--"salami science" and the "least publishable unit" and "honorary authorship." Some have argued that the few known cases of true fraud (as opposed to sloppiness or honest error) in research publishing derive from this pressure. While I would agree that the basic fault here lies with the individual who is determined to succeed at all costs, the greater fault is a system that, however unintentionally, allows irresponsibility. We are obliged to come to terms with the consequences of individual actions that bring the community's integrity into question, and to examine the system that encourages, even inadvertently, quantity over quality. It is not the pressure to publish that should concern us first, but rather the scientific community's laxness in making plain and enforcing forthrightly its own standards of work and merit. Further, we need to take seriously the fact that few senior researchers, much less their parent institutions, teach their junior colleagues the ethical standards upon which the integrity of science and scientific publishing rest.

It is not in fabrication of data that the pressure to publish hurts science most. The concern is more subtle and therefore more difficult to comprehend and address. When it leads a researcher to cut corners, diluting the value of contributions and distorting the literature, or when the tendency is to manipulate research data so that it is more tidy or less ambiguous, with the hope that such clarity will raise the chances of publication, here is a folly that does far more long-term harm. When grant or promotion committees equate quality with the number of publications, and reward researchers who work the system well because they choose fashionable topics, here is a slow-working erosion of integrity more durable than the transient bold lie. Funding institutions want more than ever to justify their choices to an increasingly critical Congress and observant citizenry. In only a few decades, many citizens have gone from being respectful supporters and grateful recipients of medical breakthroughs to being vocal, even raucous proponents of specific areas of research. This generates contradictory pressures. On the one hand, increased public scrutiny demands greater "relevance" from research for fewer dollars; while on the other, the requirement to produce results to get the dwindling resources increases competition for shrinking opportunities. Any funding committee faced with these choices wants a firm, responsible, publicly justifiable basis for its decisions. But quantity of published work cannot be the measure; to revert to a previous metaphor, it would be a debased currency.

Nevertheless, the signs are that many science researchers feel that their careers depend on publishing often, in the most prestigious journals possible, and that quantity counts more than quality. In a sense, they understand how the science community has adjusted to publication inflation. Insiders know how to read the publications lists of those within their own specialized research area-- they recognize the padding and go straight to the few publications that matter. They do not need to do this in other disciplines, and so they may feel that the system works well enough. So long as researchers can publish in ways that promote their careers, they feel pressure from the system, but many will see no inherent reason to change the standards for publication or revise the criteria for recognition and reward. In fact, the younger members and even some mid-level members of the community may feel threatened by the direction that editors' discussions and rule-setting takes.

AUTHORSHIP

What we see is an environment, in which for years (some would say decades) authorship credit on a byline has come to be the currency of this academic accounting system, taking its values not from the norms of research but from the pressures of the marketplace.[1] Regardless of how the values of the research community change or reform, researchers will pursue their place in the publication market by "authoring" as many articles as they believe are needed for their careers. Authors need to see their names attached to articles published in the journals considered important by their peers and funders. In itself, this is not a concern, but when it is at the expense of substance or integrity, then it becomes a matter of some importance to all who share in the enterprise or benefit from it. Runaway inflation is no healthier in publishing than it is in the economy at large. Therefore, the moves to limit the number of publications considered for tenure, promotion, or funding are sound and should be tried extensively. To have reservations about how the limitations will work in practice is not to doubt that the effort is worthwhile.

If authorship is seen merely as a "money of account" in this accounting system, researchers can feel free to give, trade, and buy these byline places. Further, critics will have a hard time justifying why authors should change their well-entrenched and successful habit of treating byline space as one more negotiable commodity in the academic marketplace, not essentially different from making arrangements for lab space, assistants, equipment, and the other basics of science research. This concept of byline authorship, as merely one part of the larger research enterprise, developed as science moved from the older forms of academic life (low salaries, relatively cloistered community, scholarly norms) to the new forms of academic life (being part of big business/big government/big science). Its natural expression came as projects grew so large that many authors were involved; distortion set in when researchers began to publish smaller and smaller bits of their research and yet retain the numerous authors, producing more separate titles for each author to claim.

Several decades of this practice eventually aroused concern among some in the research community, often journal editors, who found themselves confronted with the disturbing side effects.[2] As editors saw the situation, authors seemed to be publishing more and shorter articles about less and less, while at the same time the list of authors grew longer and longer. Research on publishing patterns bore out this impression. As one wry comment went, when the author list is longer than the abstract, you know you have a problem. The problem, of course, is that in most cases such an imbalance trivializes the research process.

Discussions among concerned researchers and editors gradually led to guidelines or standards that editors could agree upon in deciding who should be considered an author. Since journal editors in biomedical areas come from biomedical or academic backgrounds, they understood how distorted the system of authorship had become, and they understood the goals, values, and pressures of each group. Understanding the academic and scholarly publishing worlds, they could devise reasonable and flexible standards. The most widely cited one was written by the International Committee of Medical Journal Editors (ICJME).[3] The new guidelines immediately made a major difference because the committee members were editors of many of the most influential and well-known medical journals; they put the consensus statement into effect at their journals; and hundreds of other biomedical journals soon followed suit, although sometimes with small modifications of the basic guidelines.

These guidelines rest on the basic question of who should receive public credit for the work being reported in the article. Let us look at this issue of credit to see whether it can give us the framework we need to see the authorship question more clearly.

CREDIT

Authorship is essentially taking public credit for the work being described. By putting their names on the byline, authors are claiming due recognition for their work and accepting full responsibility for its accuracy and the integrity of its processes.

In biomedical science, teams rather than solitary researchers conduct most research. The teams may take different shapes, but they exist for well-recognized and legitimate reasons, well known to all of us. But the relationship between membership on the team and space on the byline is not always understood by the team members. To complicate matters, the different disciplines have developed separate, sometimes conflicting, informal guidelines for assigning or awarding authorship to team members. Moreover, the senior investigators seldom work out ahead of time how the article will be written, who will be responsible for what, and who will be carried on the byline. Virtually everyone in biomedical publishing knows of last-minute fallings out among authors over who should be considered an author, in what order the names should appear, and who should be credited in the acknowledgements but not on the byline.[4]

Scientists want, naturally enough, to receive appropriate credit for their work. Deciding who should usually or normally be considered an author is essentially a question of deciding who deserves credit for the article, in contrast to knowing who contributed to the research project. That is, there is a difference between being on the research project and being an author of the research article. A complete list of those involved in a research project normally contains more names than would appear on a byline.

In considering credit for an article, the senior investigator(s) must decide, first, which team members carry responsibility that entitles them to authorship credit, and, second, must agree on how the paper will be written.[5] Let us look at the ICMJE's criteria for author status. It says that authors are those who (1) conceived or designed the project, (2) executed the experiment or did the hands-on field work, (3) analyzed and interpreted the data, and (4) drafted the article or revised it critically for important intellectual content. Editors differ on how they apply these guidelines to their journals. Some may feel that a researcher should meet two of these four criteria in order to be an author; others, stricter, feel that any author must meet three. Nonetheless, the principle of assigning appropriate authorship and the role of the journal editor in setting reasonable and flexible standards are clear. The intent is equally clear: the desire to correct or at least diminish several abuses of authorship that have grown up in recent decades.

First, editors want to do away with "honorary authorship," those situations in which senior researchers pressure their junior colleagues to add the seniors' names because they head the department, laboratory, or facility involved, and want credit for the work under their general leadership. Likewise, editors want to keep ambitious junior colleagues from gratuitously adding the names of eminent seniors to their manuscripts as a way to add cachet and presumably increase their chances for publication. Senior administrators fairly often require that their names be added, whereas it is more unusual for junior members to add their senior colleagues' names without permission. Senior researchers may feel unhappy that the guidelines or standards are being changed at the time when they have reached the point in their careers in which they can benefit from the honorary authorship system. They grew up academically in a system that virtually dictated that senior administrators' names would appear on all publications. Thus, now that they have paid their dues, they feel ill-treated that they are criticized for trying to garner the very rewards that they gave their own mentors and lab chiefs over the years. In this context, their dissatisfaction is understandable. It is not a reason to soften the newly developing standards, however, for a reformed system that emphasizes quality over quantity will be able to recognize the seniors' contributions.

Second, editors and others want to limit the total number of authors for an article to those who should appropriately receive the byline credit. As article length decreases and the number of authors increases, editors want to ensure that at least the numerous names that appear are truly authors. Editors in most biomedical fields become suspicious when faced with a 2,000-word submission that carries 11 authors.

By using the ICMJE's criteria--or any other thoughtful set--editors can ask the important questions about authorship: who did the work, and who is therefore responsible for it? This brings us to the issue of taking responsibility for the work.

RESPONSIBILITY

The pernicious consequence of using authorship as a currency of exchange is that it dilutes responsibility for what is reported in the published article. When one person conducts the research and publishes the report, all readers know who is responsible for the completeness, integrity, and correctness of the report. The researcher's results may not stand up to the scrutiny of readers' and colleagues' review, but that is the way normal science works. Should the peers find the work shoddy or the report misleading, they have no doubt about who is responsible. This side of the credit-responsibility coin is important to maintaining integrity in research.

As the number of authors grows, however, the responsibility for the whole article or its parts becomes diffuse.[6] In egregious cases, some authors collect but do not analyze the data or write the paper; while their co-authors write the paper but have nothing to do with designing the experiment or handling the collected data. Who, the editor might reasonably ask, is responsible for this paper? The traditional answer is that the senior author is responsible, but troublesome cases in recent years show that some senior authors have nothing to do with the papers except that their names appear on the byline. When criticisms fly, can this senior author take responsibility for the article's contents? When finger-pointing begins, it seems that the authors all turn out to be followers and no one is leader.

At a minimum, we can expect each author to take responsibility for the article as a whole and for each to defend and confirm the part for which he or she is responsible. But recently we have seen science authors taking the credit, but not the responsibility. For example, some of John Slutsky's coauthors, although knowing that they were coauthors, said that they knew nothing about the content of the papers carrying their names and could not respond to the mounting evidence of mistakes or fraud.[7] More recently, David Baltimore retracted his authorship of the Cell article on which he shared the byline with primary investigator Thereza Imanishi-Kari.[8] The surprise is not that he did so, but that he had defended the paper and his role in it for so long.

The major ethical problem here is the uncoupling of responsibility from authorship. All biomedical editors with more than a few years' experience have seen a version of the following scenario of a problem discovered during editing. The examples are extreme but illustrate quickly the abandoning of responsibility. For example, numbers given in tables and text do not agree; or the references listed do not correlate with the citations; or, upon detailed examination, the results are not consistent with the details of the method described. (You may say, and rightly, that this indicates a problem with the review process, but that is another arena and will be put aside here.) When an editor approaches the senior or corresponding author to ask for correction or clarification of these problems, the editors can receive some strange responses: "That isn't anything I was involved in, so I can't answer you," or "The post-doc handled this and took all his notes with him when he left us three years ago; we don't know where he is," or "We lost the data but we're sure the paper is correct." In some extreme cases, there may be no collaborating data, or the sources may not say what is claimed.

There is a rather shocking insouciance here, and I have encountered authors who confess to worse than this and seem to think that they have done nothing questionable. Authors who believe that they are entitled to credit for work they took little part in, perhaps do not understand, cannot explain, or much less defend are breaking faith with their peers. The authors in the scenario, albeit extreme examples, illustrate more clearly than usual the problem of taking credit but shirking responsibility. As Patricia Woolf reminded us at the 1988 Council of Biology of Editors conference on ethics in biomedical publishing, moral responsibility cannot be divided, for there is no such thing as division of moral labor.[9] Certainly, research teams can decide among themselves how to divide the physical labor of conducting, analyzing, and writing up their research, but they should not think that they can divide up the moral responsibility for the accuracy and correctness of the published work that carries their name.

This is so because scientific teamwork must be based on trust, and acceptance of the research is most often an act of faith. Team members must trust that their specialist colleagues use appropriate measures, accurate techniques, and tell the truth when collecting data and analyzing it. In teams, they must accept as a given that their colleagues are doing what they say they are doing--if the preliminary results are supposedly based on the review of 55 medical charts, appropriately selected according to an agreed-upon protocol, the team assumes as a matter of trust that the colleagues responsible for the review actually reviewed the charts and collected the correct information. The "gentleman's agreement" in science is left over from the days when "gentleman scientists" pursued learning for its own sake and had little reason to lie other than vainglory. Today, when science is big business, the reasons to cheat begin at vanity, but quickly go on to encompass ambition in the form of grant money, tenure, speaking invitations, and the rewards of renown. Yet, although science is now a major industry, trustworthiness remains central; it is the weight-bearing member of the scientific edifice. In conducting research, the scientist combines this essential trust of colleagues' integrity with a healthy skepticism about the research being done.

But this sturdy skepticism that lies at the heart of well-conducted science has generally not been applied to the workings of large research teams. Most of us are now amused to hear the story of Henry Stimson, US Secretary of State under Herbert Hoover, who refused to let British Intelligence and the FBI intercept prominent German nationals' mail in the United States because "gentlemen don't read other gentlemen's mail." Senior intelligence operatives were not so amused, and neither should the research community be when the principle is applied to research teams. The conclusion that researchers should not question team members' work abandons all the proper scientific skepticism at one of the crucial parts of research. The absurd and pernicious outcome of honorary authorship is that a person who has not done the research and in some cases has not even read the paper will be carried as an author of a published scientific report and therefore accept public responsibility for its accuracy.

Editors' concerns about appropriate authorship should not be seen as the suspicions of the muck raker or (as Drummond Rennie[10] cast us editors) mark, dupe, patsy, accessory, weasel, or flatfoot. Rather, editors' concerns should be accepted as science's ordinary and necessary skepticism applied to publishing just as it is to experimental study. When editors ask authors, as they increasingly do, to complete and sign a document that explains the contribution that each made to the article being submitted, the editors are not "gentlemen reading other gentlemen's mail." Instead, they are raising a normal issue for science: show me that this is so. In this case, a group of people claim that they are authors of the paper according to the criteria the journal has laid down for authorship, and the editor asks that they spell out their contributions so that the connection between each person's work and the finished article will be explicit.

These documents are the concrete expression of the continuing debate over authorship for scientific publishing. That editors need such forms shows how far the concepts of credit and responsibility have drifted in scientific papers. We can hope that using sound authorship criteria will again mean that authors who claim credit on article bylines are ready to accept public responsibility for the articles that appear under their name.

REFLECTIONS

In theory, authors and editors have the same goals in scholarly publishing: to communicate valid and useful information within the scholarly community, and to improve society, even if indirectly. But just as drivers and pedestrians usually have different opinions about traffic and driving conditions during city rush hours, authors and editors often hold strikingly divergent views on the proper values and procedures for science publishing. A perennial problem that highlights their differences is the issue of authorship. The specifics can seem trivial: a journal limits to six the number of authors allowed for a research report; laboratory directors or senior administrators expect to be carried as authors for any paper written in units they supervise, whether or not they were involved in the project; the skilled technicians who conduct the day-to-day work upon which the report is based feel that their contribution warrants authorship credit; and when published results are questioned, some of the listed authors respond that their involvement in the project was too limited for them to be held accountable for their coauthors' mistakes or misconduct.

In biomedical publishing, these are not trivial problems; instead, they lie at the heart of the scientific community's struggle to conduct productive research and communicate it. The issue is two-sided: authors should receive appropriate credit in publishing, and they should take responsibility for what they publish. Seen in this context, the apparently trivial questions of how many authors should be allowed on one article and how they are to be chosen and listed, or the issue of authors being held accountable for an article's accuracy, are certainly central to the scientific endeavor. The Western scientific tradition is based on trust and mutual responsibilities, but within research teams and between editor and authors, this trust must be tempered by scientific skepticism. In the biomedical community, the responsibilities take on additional importance, for the communication extends to the patient's bedside, where physicians and others apply directly the information they learn from colleagues' articles.

When science was a smaller enterprise, the rules could be those of a gentleman's agreement--scientists did not lie, and their goal was held to be a greater good that usually brought no direct benefit to them other than fame within their group, and seldom led to wealth or even remuneration. (This is the idealized sketch, of course, for scoundrels and cheats turned up in this system; there was fairly clear agreement, however, on what constituted a cheat, and they were summarily excluded from science's inner circle by group pressure.)

Modern-day science, however, is one of the largest components of industrial society, usually linked to big government and often to big business. As science has assumed more of the forms of commercial or bureaucratic life, so have its gentleman's rules proved inadequate to the intense national and international competition among the burgeoning ranks of scientists. Tens of thousands of researchers compete for the resources to conduct research and report results that will bring, at the least, continued support and, sometimes, wealth and worldwide fame. Societies eventually regulate any enterprise that proves vital to their well-being. We are not surprised that government now controls stock markets, that nations control fishing in international waters, or that the international community tries to control even war with rules of behavior. Why should anyone be surprised that society expects controls on the products of science and even its mechanisms? So far, this control is still internal to the community, in that journal editors and leading scientists are trying to frame criteria that will maintain high standards for authorship (and through that mechanism, for the rewards that flow from authorship). Thus, editors have begun to spell out increasingly specific rules for publishing that will limit the problems and protect the usefulness of biomedical publishing. By working out these standards and guidelines, discussing them in conferences of editors and authors, and promulgating them as basic tenets of the operation of scientific research, editors have moved a long way toward setting consensus standards for research publishing. Now the research community and editors must continue working together to test these standards, refine them as needed, and thereby support the integrity of science publishing.

NOTES

1   W.B. Frye, "Medical Authorship: Traditions, Trends, and Tribulations, *Annals of Internal Medicine* 113 (1990):317-25; D.P. Carrigan, "Publish or Perish: The Troubled State of Scholarly Communication, *Scholarly Publishing* 22, no.3 (1991):131-42.
2   E.J. Huth, "Editors and the Problems of Authorship: Rulemakers or Gatekeepers?" in *Ethics and Policy in Scientific Publication* (Bethesda, MD: Council of Biology Editors, 1990), 175-80; E.J. Huth, *Scientific Authorship and Publication: Process, Standards, Problems, Suggestions* (Washington, DC: Institute of Medicine, National Academy of Sciences, 1988); E.J. Huth, "Irresponsible Authorship and Wasteful Publication," *Annals of Internal Medicine* 104 (1986):257-59; P.P. Morgan, "How Many Authors Can Dance on the Head of an Article?" *Canadian Medical Association Journal* 130 (1984):842.
3   International Committee of Medical Journal Editors, "Uniform Requirements for Manuscripts Submitted to Biomedical Journals," *New England Journal of Medicine* 324 (1991):424-28.
4   International Committee of Medical Journal Editors, "Statements from the International Committee of Medical Journal Editors ['Order of Authorship']," *Journal of the American Medical Association* 265 (1991):2697-98.
5   V.N. Houk and S.B. Thacker, "The Responsibilities of Scientific Authorship," in *Ethics and Policy in Scientific Publication* (Bethesda, MD: Council of Biology Editors, 1990), 181-84, reprinted in *Scholarly Publishing* 22, no.1 (1991):51-55; E.J. Huth, "Guidelines on Authorship of Medical Papers," *Annals of Internal Medicine* 104 (1986):269-74; Morgan, "How Many Authors?"
6   D. Kennedy, "Accountability and Authorship," in *Ethics and Policy in Scientific Publication* (Bethesda, MD: Council of Biology Editors, 1991), 115-23.
7   R.L. Engler, J.W. Covell, and P.J. Friedman, "Misrepresentation and Re-

sponsibility in Medical Research," *New England Journal of Medicine* 317 (1987): 1383-89; P.J. Friedman, "Correcting the Literature Following Fraudulent Publication," *Journal of the American Medical Association* 263 (1990):1416-19.

8   D. Weaver, M.H. Reis, C. Albanese, *et al.*, "Altered Repertoire of Endogenous Immunoglobulin Gene Expression in Transgenic Mice Containing a Rearranged *mu* Heavy Chain Gene," *Cell* 45, no.2 (1986):247-59, article retracted by four of its five authors, May 1991.

9   P. Woolf, "Open Discussion [of 'Accountability and Authorship: Where Does the Responsibility Lie?'']," in *Ethics and Policy in Scientific Publication* (Bethesda, MD: Council of Biology Editors, 1990), 125.

10   D. Rennie, "The Editor: Mark, Dupe, Patsy, Accessory, Weasel, and Flatfoot," in *Ethics and Policy in Scientific Publication* (Bethesda, MD: Council of Biology Editors, 1990):155-67.

7

Uses and Abuses of Scientific Authorship: Can and Should They Be Controlled?

Edward J. Huth

I like the title of a recently published book, *Toward the Habit of Truth: A Life in Science,* by Mahlon Hoagland, the eminent molecular biologist.[1] The text features his reflections on the people, practices, and politics of scientific work. As one reviewer of this book summarized, it is the phrase "the habit of truth" that carries the essence of what should govern the conduct of science. But even if all who work in science were to agree with this sentiment, there are many points in science at which "truth" has to be defined. What is the meaning of "authorship" for both writers and readers of scientific literature?

THE FRAME THROUGH WHICH TO EXAMINE AUTHORSHIP

Why should the topic of authorship be in the agenda of a symposium on scientific conduct? Perhaps the organizers have seen this function as falling short of standards for the proper conduct of science--to a degree and frequency that is likely to damage science. And behind this premise must be a preceding one that science is a function in our society with values for us worth saving. Notice that I use terms like "damage" and "worth" and "values," rather than "unethical" and "ethical." This choice is deliberate. I must make clear that I prefer to see ethical issues not as dealing with alternative categories such as "good" and "bad" or even the softer "ethical" and "unethical." I see the issues, rather, in economic terms, as conflicts of economic needs. In this phrase, I include power and other resources that can be applied to serving economic needs; as a result, the term "economic" is broader than merely referring to financial matters. To avoid analyzing my view at a length that is inappropriate here, let me state simply that I do not believe that persons who deviate from the standards of authorship desire to see themselves as "unethical" or "bad"; instead, they are placing their personal economic needs ahead of the economic needs of science.

What does science expect of its authors? For most of the roughly 400 years during which science has been striving to identify the right questions and their correct answers, it has asked (mainly of authors) that they be honest, that their written words be regarded as reliable. This need is an economic need; scientists desiring to move forward by answering new questions do not wish to risk wasting their resources--time, work, funds--in trying to build new evidence on false foundations. So the name of the author on a paper has been taken to mean that this person affirms the reliability of what the paper says. On the author's side was the economic gain from honesty. Indeed, when authors produced reliable fact and concept on which others could build, they were likely to achieve high economic rewards, including further support from patrons, appointments to higher posts with better returns, and more power to engage in more science. Thus, authors who were sole authors took both responsibility for what they wrote and credit for its values. Responsibility was what the author owed science; credit was the payback from science.

Science has become more complex. As experiments and observations came to involve more and more difficult methods, and more and more subjects in particular studies, the numbers of persons engaged per piece of scientific work began to increase. With this change came a climb in the average number of authors per paper.[2] As lists of authors in papers have lengthened, questions about their functions as authors have begun to arise. Consider today's elaborate multicenter clinical trials of treatments for cancer or for coronary artery disease: If one includes not only the so-called principal investigators, but also persons gathering data from, or caring for, patients, the numbers can reach into the hundreds. Who among these increasing numbers of persons engaged per piece of work should be identified as authors on the resulting papers? This question cannot be answered without first defining "author."

DEFINITIONS OF AUTHORSHIP

Some scholarly groups and editors have developed and published definitions of scientific authorship.[3] Their views generally stem from the concept of an author as a person who takes responsibility for the content of a paper, who accepts as a duty what science expects of an author. Taking responsibility is more than simply affirming the truth and correctness of a paper's content; it includes having the capacity to defend the content of the paper if it is questioned after publication. If an investigator takes the position of author, then what part must he or she have had in the reported work, and what are the author's responsibilities? The most explicit of definitions representing a consensus defines the needed author's participation as:

Each author should have participated sufficiently in the work to take public responsibility for the content. Authorship credit should be based only on substantial contributions to (a) conception and design, or analysis and interpretation of data, and to (b) drafting the article or revising it critically for important intellectual content; and on (c) final approval of the version to be published. Conditions (a), (b), and (c) must all be met. Participation solely in the acquisition of funding or the collection of data does not justify authorship. General supervision of the research group is also not sufficient for authorship.[4]

This definition goes on to require that a paper carry as authors all persons thus definable, so that all of the paper's content is represented by a responsible person: "Any part of an article critical to its main conclusions must be the responsibility of at least one author."

The authors are responsible for appointing authorship, but "editors may require authors to justify the assignment of authorship." This collective judgment of the editors comprising the International Committee of Medical Journal Editors has been elaborated on for both clinical papers[5] and for a particular research center;[6] the second of these elaborations presents an even more detailed analysis and definition.

Little published and formal analysis of proper criteria for authorship has come from authors; their views have been represented mainly in "letters to the editor" prompted by papers such as that cited above.[7] Their views have tended to emphasize the importance of public credit to participants; the most recent extended statement of this kind acknowledges the central importance of responsibility, but calls for more prominent statements of credit in published papers.[8] The concept of credit may be no less complex than that of what represents the capacity to accept responsibility as an author. Should credit simply represent a statement of work done? Or is this definition likely to dilute (or cheapen) the concept of "credit" as a "post hoc" judgment of science that develops well after a paper appears, and only after the paper's validity and importance have been supported by replicating studies or by testing what it implies for study of new questions?

Some authors complain that editors are offensively parsimonious with the kind of definition of authorship illustrated above. They point to the need for young scientists to get visibility for their work. They argue that restricting authorship damages developing careers. But they may not see that gratuitous, or marginally justified, authorship cheapens the value of authorship: a kind of Gresham's law of scientific literature. Those who argue for a less restrictive definition should consider that they are likely to have to judge, at some future time, a candidate for appointment or tenure. They may then find themselves baffled by the task of determining the degree to which the candidate truly contributed to the science that is represented by a long list of papers carrying his or her name in various positions within lengthy author lists.

WHERE SHOULD AUTHORSHIP BE JUDGED?

Editors have led, at least in medicine, in defining authorship. But they have been reluctant to impose arbitrary judgments on authorship of papers they publish. This reluctance is reasonable. There are no simple means by which they can judge the validity of authorship of a particular paper, even with a clear definition in hand. The number of authors on a paper is, itself, usually no clue to inappropriate authorship. Now and then, the content of a paper suggests that the number of "authors" is excessive, such as a report of a single and essentially simple case. But for papers with complex content, or based on large and complex studies, a large number of authors may be entirely justified. Indeed, in at least one field, high-energy particle physics, a large number of authors on a single paper (for example, 200) may look like a gross abuse of authorship to readers accustomed to papers with 10 authors or fewer. But an experiment in particle physics may depend on being able to detect subatomic "events" with a vast and costly custom-built piece of apparatus developed out of a concept specific to the experiment. The experiment may need weeks of continuous data collection, constantly monitored. The analysis of the data may itself intellectually challenge even those who designed the experiment. Who can judge, simply from reading the paper, whether all 200 "authors" met a clear definition of author?

Sometimes editors can have their doubts about the legitimacy of authorship when they see disparities between a paper's content and the number of investigators one can suppose would have been needed to generate it. This is why the definition of authorship quoted above goes on to say that editors can ask for justifications. But even if they are asked for and supplied, the editor still must trust the stated authors to take responsibility for the legitimacy of the stated authorship.

Ultimately, the defining of authorship and honest use of that definition are the duty of the scientists who accept authorship. This is a duty to their profession and to themselves as representatives of it. The right definition and the right use of it must be part of the ethos of science, must be a readily, preferably unconsciously, applied rule of conduct. In recent years, we have seen plenty of evidence that science can fall short of this standard, even science in institutions of high repute. Consider, for example, the following cases.

Some multi-authored papers on a genetic aspect of gastrointestinal disease are suspected of presenting fraudulent data. After the author who is believed to have committed the fraud admits to it, his coauthors issued statements that they repudiate the papers' content, that they had nothing to do with the fraud.

One must ask, why these coauthors accepted authorship when they had been so unconnected with the gathering of the evidence presented in the papers that they could not vouch for its validity? Their proper response to the uncovering of fraud should have been a statement that they accepted authorship without having an adequate basis for it.

In a closely related second case, involving a different university, experimental data were forged by the author responsible for the fraud in the first. After several investigations in different institutions, he admitted to committing this second fraud. Another of the authors on this paper, a man highly eminent in his field, engaged lawyers who tried through intimidation to block publication of a scholarly and analytical paper that suggested he might not have been involved enough in the experimental work to be able to vouch for its authenticity.

Why did he not simply prepare himself to admit that he might not have been sufficiently involved in the reported experiment to ensure the authenticity of the data? He could have gained in stature through being willing to concede poor judgment.

These are not recent cases, but in reviewing them now I have come to feel that the definition of authorship quoted above may not be fully adequate; perhaps it should explicitly include sufficient participation in the gathering of evidence to satisfy oneself, as an author, that the evidence is authentic. This requirement, I admit, may be too demanding; certainly in large multicenter clinical trials the responsible investigators cannot be on hand for the collecting of each and every datum that makes up the evidence. Such obstacles suggest that the ground rules for the writing and publishing of multi-authored papers should require that the original materials for the evidence be filed in an institutional archive so that any one of the authors could at any time, before or after publication, review them for assurance of their authenticity.

WHAT CAN BE DONE TO KEEP AUTHENTIC AUTHORSHIP IN THE ETHOS OF SCIENCE?

As illustrated above, some scholarly organizations in science and some scientific editors have defined authorship. Yet there is much evidence that the definitions are not widely known among potential authors. Some of this fault lies with editors. There are journals that explicitly define authorship in their information-for-authors pages. But many publications do not provide such guidelines, even some journals subscribing to the Uniform Requirements document quoted above.[9] Who is going to push these journals into defining authorship for their potential authors? This is a task that could be assumed by societies of editors, such as those now representing the biological sciences and the earth sciences in the United States and in Europe. But such definitions are generally remote in both location and consciousness from where papers are written and authorship accepted--the sites where the science is carried on. I see the need for academic centers and research institutes to establish their own definitions of authorship, or affirm those published, and to establish means to try to ensure that they are properly applied. Some efforts of this kind have already led to means for dealing with questions of conflict of interest and of fraud; surely their scope could be widened to deal with questions of authorship. Local attention to authorship can raise awareness of the need to agree on a proper definition; one of the authors whose paper[10] is cited above has assured[11] many of us in the editorial business that such attention can reduce disputes about authorship, and I am ready to believe that it can support authentic authorship.

But while we wait for the academic world to set its standards for authorship, we should expect editors of medical journals to do what they can to influence the ethos of medical science. What can they do? Medical editors can publish clear statements in their journals of how they define legitimate authorship. Editors can expect authors to sign statements affirming the legitimacy of their authorship, as judged by the criteria set by the journal. In cases of disputed authorship that cannot be settled by the putative authors, an editor can inform the disputing potential authors that without a solution by them he or she will turn to their academic superiors for a solution. Finally, editors should be expected to support a desirable ethos for research by publishing notices of retraction of flawed work and letters bearing on disputes of authorship.

I am sure that American science does not wish to have its work scrutinized and regulated by a Washington-based commissar of science, but that is what might result if medical research does not establish its own and effective ethos for honest reporting. And in the locales of science there can be legitimate objections to yet more administrative manipulation, even that locally based. Yet in the wider society of American life, the mere existence of courts, which can impose penalties, likely deters some misconduct and thereby supports an ethos of values that are used by citizens to guide their day-to-day activities at work and within the community. How more academic communities and research institutes can be persuaded to find practical ways to encourage in their own places the "habit of truth," I do not know.

To answer the question in my title: Yes, uses and abuses of authorship should be controlled; science owes this to itself for its good health. But the control should be of a kind that comes easily--out of the proper habits of responsibility of scientists to one other, and out of an ethos accepted and respected by all.

NOTES

1   M. Hoagland, *Toward the Habit of Truth: A Life in Science* (New York: Norton, 1990).

2   E.J. Huth, "Editors and the Problems of Authorship: Rulemakers or Gatekeepers?" in *Ethics and Policy in Scientific Publication* (Bethesda, MD: Council of Biology Editors, 1990), 175-80.

3   *Ibid.*

4   International Committee of Medical Journal Editors (ICMJE), "Uniform Requirements for Manuscripts Submitted to Biomedical Journals," *New England Journal of Medicine* 324 (1991):424-28.

5   E.J. Huth, "Guidelines on Authorship of Medical Papers," *Annals of Internal Medicine* 104 (1986): 269-74.
6   ICMJE, "Uniform Requirements."
7   C.C. Conrad, "Authorship, Acknowledgment, and Other Credit," in *Ethics and Policy in Scientific Publication* (Bethesda, MD: Council of Biology Editors, 1990), 184-87.
8   ICMJE, "Uniform Requirements."
9   V.N. Houk and S.B. Thacker, "The Responsibilities of Authorship," in *Ethics and Policy in Scientific Publication* (Bethesda, MD: Council of Biology Editors, 1990), 181-84.
10 V.N. Houk, "Discussion," in *Ethics and Policy in Scientific Publication* (Bethesda, MD: Council of Biology Editors, 1990), 196.

8

Is Being an Author the Key to Success?

Sharon G. Boots

Although present-day journals can be traced to the late 16th and early 17th centuries,[1] the time of the first scientific revolution, the world's most prestigious medical and chemical journals[2] had their beginnings in the late 1800s. What were the transportation and communication systems like at this time and how did these influence interactions among scholars?

During the 1870s, Alexander Graham Bell, a teacher of the deaf in Boston, experimented at night with a harmonic telegraph. One of the metal reeds stuck. His assistant, Thomas Watson, snapped the reed to loosen it, causing vibrations which, in turn, caused variations in the electric current that Bell picked up in his receiver in the next room. The rest is history; and, in 1876, Bell and Watson held the first two-way long distance phone conversation between Boston and Cambridge, a distance of two miles. In 1892, service began between New York and Chicago. The 1949 invention of the transistor made it possible to effectively use undersea telephone cables. Telephone service began operating between Europe and the United States in 1956, and between Japan and the US in 1964.

What were transportation systems like? By the end of the 1800s the US had five transcontinental rail lines. The first was completed in 1869. In 1893-1894, Charles E. and J. Frank Duryea built the first successful American gasoline-powered car. In 1903, the Winton traveled coast to coast in 63 days. In the same year, Orville and Wilbur Wright made history near Kitty Hawk, North Carolina. During the early 1920s, several small passenger airlines were started in the US. In 1935, the US had four major domestic airlines, and by the late 1930s, the world's airlines carried 3.5 million passengers. During the late 1800s, the primary purpose of scientific publications was to communicate scientific information. And by 1850 there were a few thousand scientific journals. As travel became easier and faster, scientific meetings became an increasingly important way for scientists to share information. Later, more advanced communications systems (for example, sophisticated telephones and facsimile machines, and the networks such as Internet and Bitnet) sped the flow of scientific ideas. Access to people and information, cross-fertilization of ideas, and networking became easier. Today, meeting organizers publish abstracts, preprints, proceedings, and even full-length papers close to the time of the meeting. The telephone, preprint distribution, and oral presentations, and the ensuing publications have largely supplanted the original intent of journals--to disseminate original and unique scientific information. You may ask, then, why do we need paper journals today? Primarily because the most prestigious paper journals have always served an archival purpose and will probably continue to do so. This is our written record of scientific progress. In addition, journals were the primary way that scientists communicated; consequently, most journal articles contained extensive experimental details and balanced discussion sections. Scientists considered themselves scholars and published their research findings in scholarly journals. Because there were so few other formal means of communication, journals filled a unique niche in the late 1800s-early 1900s; they continue to play an important role despite the many other ways used to communicate science. The most elite journals (*New England Journal of Medicine, Journal of the American Medical Association, Science,* and *Nature,* to name a few) have become known today as the purveyors of "reliable" scientific information--reliable in the sense that only accurate articles, which have been scrutinized carefully by the experts (peer reviewed), are published.

As a contrast, conference abstracts, proceedings, and preprints are generally not peer reviewed in depth (often not at all), are likely to be uneven in quality, and do not necessarily contain the detailed experimental and discussion sections found in full-length journal articles. In an effort to describe the most recent data, many speakers discuss experiments performed the week before or even a few hours before the talk. Many abstracts are prepared long before the meeting and contain a discussion of results that the authors hope to substantiate by the time of the meeting. In addition, many meeting organizers are not selective in choosing speakers for their programs, and anyone can submit an abstract and present a paper. Many scientists view the material found in these publications as preliminary accounts of research and often regard them with suspicion: "Let the reader beware." What has happened to the numbers of published journals as other means of communication have become increasingly important? The rise in the number of journals has been dramatic--Ulrich's database lists approximately 120 thousand journals in all fields and over 74 thousand science and technology titles.[3] Over 29 thousand science titles were added between 1978 and 1987.[4]

Although there is some indication that the rate of increase has diminished, why has the number of journals increased at such an astounding rate? Is this growth good or bad? Does it merely indicate a growth in the productivity of the scientific community or are other factors at work as well? Much of science has become "big business." To be a successful scientist and run a productive research program in today's environment, one not only must be creative, but also an entrepreneur. One must be savvy in how to obtain funds and write grant proposals that succeed, as well as be able to identify areas of research that are likely to be funded. One must learn how to take advantage of the system.

Publications play a key role. Raises, tenure, and promotion are primarily dependent on research and publications. Often the number of journal articles count. It has been suggested that granting agencies and tenure committees tend to judge productivity by the number of publications in peer-reviewed journals,[5] although there is movement toward examining a limited number of articles.[6] Much has been written about how authors inflate their publication lists[7]--often referred to in such terms as "duplicate publication" and "salami science." Authors have resorted to tactics such as sending essentially the same article to several journals, fragmenting their work in such a way that they report only small pieces of the entire work at a time (often referred to as the LPU or least publishable unit), and publishing just plain trivia.[8] Also, scientists have advanced their careers and inflated their publications list by allowing their names to be attached to publications as authors (honorary authorship) even though they have not been intimately involved in the work, leaving them unable to accept responsibility for the content of the paper.[9] Commercial publishers and societies alike have capitalized on scientists' desire to gain recognition by having a long publication lists. New societies envisage journal publication as a way to cement the bond among the community, and also to announce to the world that the organization has now become established and recognized. Related to this, and probably no less important, is the inclusion of the new journal into the databases of the secondary services. Commercial publishers have been quick to move into these new, emerging areas with or without the cooperation of societies and have attempted to capture papers from the more well-established, elite, broad-based journals by publishing specialty journals. However, these new journals often act as siphons, siphoning off the rejected papers from the more elite journals.

Recently, articles appeared in *Science*[10] involving the use of data from the Institute for Scientific Information's (ISI) database of scientific citations to support the idea that we are publishing way too much, and that much of it is trivial. David Pendlebury, an ISI analyst, compiled data that indicated 55 percent of the papers indexed in ISI's databases and published between 1981 and 1985 received no citations in the first five years after they appeared. ISI's database covers only the top science and social science journals--some four thousand five hundred out of nearly seventy-four thousand science and technology titles listed in the *Ulrich's* database. Self-citation (the author cites his or her own work) usually accounts for between 5 to 20 percent of all citations. Pendlebury showed that there is a wide variation among disciplines which, however, may simply indicate that fields differ in their natural expression of the creation and dissemination of knowledge. Also, different types of published items vary widely in their "uncitedness." An American Psychological Association (APA) study in 1970 determined that no paper in any core journal would be read by more than 7 percent of its readers.[11]

However, the climate is changing. NSF and NIH have limited the number of publications that can be listed in the bibliography of a grant application. Renewal applications must contain a list of all publications resulting from direct support. At this time, the Harvard Medical School guidelines recommend that the number of publications reviewed for faculty appointment or promotion be limited to between five to ten, and it appears that others will soon follow.[12] Change often appears to be slow, however; in this case, is it perhaps that numbers provide an easy yardstick? Would tenure committees be forced to do a more thorough job of critiquing the actual contributions of the individual if they only had five to ten papers to comment on? Would this actually make their evaluations easier and less time-consuming or vise versa?

Perhaps the importance attached to the numbers of publications has become firmly entrenched in science. And the current leaders, having most probably risen to the top in this way, are possibly reluctant to change. However, if the system is to change, these senior scientists, the mentors of our young people, must squarely address this issue and stress quality and not quantity in research and publications. Most agree that one yardstick for assessing quality is the use of citation data. There are those, however, who argue that less-quantitative measures provide the most meaningful information.

Also, in the past there have been few rewards at major research universities for excellence in teaching. This also is beginning to change: Stanford University has recently emphasized the importance of teaching. Others need to take a proactive role and follow this path.

A recent issue of *Sierra* (the publication of the Sierra Club) included an ad for an "Anti-Junk Mail Kit." For only $6.75 one could attempt to have one's name removed from mailing lists. The ad stated that, in 1990, 34 million trees were sacrificed for junk mail alone. This made me wonder how many trees were required to produce the paper necessary to publish unnecessary journals. Taking this one step further, of course, raises the question, are we being good stewards of the earth by encouraging the proliferation of paper journals? A recent discussion of the impact of science publishing on the environment emphasized the benefits of using recycled paper, in addition to working with a printer who is committed to avoiding waste and recycling as many materials as possible.[13]

How many journals are really necessary? Some have made educated guesses that 90 percent of the information necessary for the advancement of scientific thought appears in 10 percent of the publications. The rest is buried so deeply in the proverbial haystack that it is next to impossible to find. These journals not only cost exorbitant sums of money (resources) and overburden the already overburdened publishing enterprise, but also force scientists who want to keep abreast of the literature to make educated guesses as to where the important science is actually appearing.

The majority of journals depend heavily on institutional subscribers (libraries) for revenue. Excluded from this group are the relatively few first-tier publications that also depend heavily on advertising revenue (such as those journals mentioned earlier) and the controlled-circulation magazines that depend entirely on advertising income for revenue.

Starting a new publication is a business decision. Continuing a publication is a business decision. Commercial and nonprofit publishers alike expect to lose money on a new publication for only three to five years. After this time, they expect to make money, usually substantial amounts. Otherwise, the publication has a short life. Also, the more mature publications must continue to be financially viable or they risk being discontinued by the publisher.

Libraries play a key role. The average member of the Association of Research Libraries holds about 26 percent of those titles available. Recently, however, substantial cutbacks in library budgets have forced librarians to cancel subscriptions and take an even closer look at their holdings.

Commercial publishers often set high subscription prices that are beyond the reach of individual subscribers; therefore, many journals are almost entirely dependent on institutional subscribers for income. Such journals maintain their profitability by increasing subscription prices, sometimes by more than 50 percent in one year.[14] Journals from the major science and technology publishers have been doubling in size in approximately eleven to twelve years, and doubling in price in approximately five to six years.[15]

Libraries must continue to take a good hard look at their holdings. User surveys and university faculty evaluations of titles should be performed to identify those journals of high value. The quantity is huge. It has been estimated that one year's worth of journals indexed in MEDLINE is equivalent to twice the height of the Washington monument.[16] Again, the scientific community needs to take a proactive role and provide librarians with the information they need to make the most efficient use of allocated funds without compromising their information services.

As we move into the age of the network medium, it is tempting to allow everyone to communicate anything. Should we have the same types of restrictions as for authorship? Will the electronic system soon be burdened with so much reporting of scholarly endeavors that the "needle in the haystack" effect, so evident in the paper journals, will make it difficult to identify the sought-after articles?

For the most part, the relatively uncomplicated days of the scientist at the turn of the century are gone; uncomplicated in the sense that scientific inquiry and creativity did not necessarily depend on the scientist's entrepreneurial abilities. However, much can be done to tip the scale back toward scholarship, responsibility, and accountability. The scientific community itself must place more weight on quality--in research and in publications. The scientific community should discuss ways to assess and define quality. Less importance should be attached to long publication lists and success should be judged in a different way. In addition to (or even instead of) being judged by what one has done, one should be judged by what one has been--responsible, accountable, and honest in the pursuit of scientific inquiry.

NOTES

1   D.A. Kronick, *A History of Scientific & Technical Periodicals: The Origins and Development of the Scientific and Technical Press 1665-1790* (Metuchen, NJ: Scarecrow Press, 1976).

2   For a description of the history of chemical journals, see H. Skolnik and K.M. Reese, eds., *A Century of Chemistry* (Washington, DC: American Chemical Society, 1976). In addition, a historical presentation of the Royal Society's publication is presented by M.F. Katzen, "The Changing Appearance of Research Journals in Science and Technology: An Analysis and a Case Study," in *Development of Science Publishing in Europe*, ed. A.J. Meadows (Amsterdam: Elsevier, 1980). Another analysis is given by B. Houghton, *Scientific Periodicals; Their Historical Development, Characteristics and Control* (Linnet Books & Clive Bingley, 1975).

3   *Ulrich's International Periodicals Directory, 1990-1991*, 29th ed. (New York: Bowker, 1990).

4   "Serial Trends: Scientific Publishing Boom," *Ulrich's News* 1, no.3 (April 1988).

5   T.P. Stossel, "Volume: Papers and Academic Promotion," *Annals of Internal Medicine* 106 (1986):146-149; R.G. Petersdorf, "The Pathogenesis of Fraud in Medical Science," *Annals of Internal Medicine* 104 (1986):252-54.

6   M. Angell, "Editors and Fraud," *Council of Biology Editors Views* 6 (1983):3-8; M. Angell, "Publish or Perish: A Proposal," *Annals of Internal Medicine* 104 (1986):261-62.

7   For an excellent discussion of all aspects of authorship, see J.C. Bailar III, M. Angell, and S. Boots, *Ethics and Policy in Scientific Publication* (Bethesda, MD: Council of Biology Editors, 1990).

8   W.J. Broad, "The Publishing Game: Getting More for Less," *Science* 211 (1981):1137-39.

9   E.J. Huth, "Scientific Authorship and Publication: Process, Standards, Problems, Suggestions," a background paper for the Institute of Medicine Committee on the Responsible Conduct of Research, 1988. This paper gives an excellent overview of the types of authorship in addition to an in-depth discussion of the ethics and responsibilities involved in authorship.

10   David Hamilton has reported on this in *Science*. See, for example, "News & Comment," *Science* (7 December 1990):1331 and "News & Comment," *Science* (4 January 1991):25; these were followed by several "Letters," *Science* (22 March 1991):1408-11.

11   B. Houghton, citing H. Wooster, "The Future of Scientific Publishing," *Journal of the Washington Academy of Sciences* 60 (June 1970): 41-45.

12   Both NSF and NIH have limited the number of publications that can be listed in the bibliography when submitting grant applications. NSF asks authors to list five publications directly related to the work described in the application, and five others (*Grants for Research and Education in Science and Engineering: An Application Guide*, August 1990) whereas NIH limits it to a total of ten (PHS-398 Kit, 1991).

13   An excellent discussion of the environmental impact of science publishing was carried out at the 1991 Council of Biology Editors annual meeting, moderated by C. Kalina of the National Library of Medicine. A report of this was recently published, C. Kalina, D. Assmann, E.D. Junkin, *et al.* "The Environmental Impact of Science Publishing: Global Issues and Close to Home: What Can CBE Members Do to Minimize the Environmental Impact of Publishing?" *CBE Views* 15 (1992): 3-4.

14   J. Saylor, unpublished manuscript, "User Survey-Engineering Library," Cornell University, 1991.

15   C. Hamaker, "Journal Prices in Perspective," *ARL* 153 (7 November 1990): 1-2.

16   A. Okerson, "The Future of Journals: The Twilight of the Journal?" unpublished manuscript, University of Chicago, April 1992. In this excellent discourse of the future of journals, Okerson refers to the Spring 1990 meeting of the Association of Research Libraries where "Nancy Eaton, Director of University Libraries of Iowa State University projected a chart that had been prepared a couple of years earlier during her directorship at the University of Vermont Libraries. In that chart, the Washington Monument stood shoulder high to the pile of journals indexed by Medline. A study done by Chuck Hamaker of Louisiana State University (described in ARL's newsletter issue no. 153) suggests that if one considers number of issues to be a surrogate for journal size growth, then the output of the largest STM publishers' journals double in size in 10-12 years. At that rate of growth, the Medline stack would indeed equal two Washington Monuments in 1992."

9

Misrepresentation of Data and Other Misconduct in Science: The German View and Experience

Albin Eser

In the same way that research is not bound to national borders, the phenomenon of "misconduct in science" is not limited to the United States. Though misconduct of researchers in the US has been given more attention so far, eventually it will be found also in Western Europe, and probably elsewhere, too.

However, misconduct in science is international in other senses as well. Very often it may be necessary to go beyond borders when individual complaints of misconduct have to be investigated; for example, in a case in which a researcher has continued or even started the misconduct during a research stay abroad.[1] Or there may also be international implications in cases where falsified research results have been published in a foreign journal. Such examples likely represent the majority of serious cases of misconduct by researchers from non-English-speaking countries, because most scientific journals of international rank are published in the United States or Great Britain.[2]

It is quite obvious that international problems of this sort cannot be solved on a purely national level; therefore, a border-crossing approach is needed. The approach must represent more or less uniform rules of conduct for researchers, and for dealing with cases of misconduct (hopefully on a worldwide scale); and it must give due regard to national peculiarities. It is also obvious, however, that there is still a long way to go, especially considering that in many countries there is no national-level consensus on the correct way in which to treat misconduct

For assistance in preparing this contribution I am greatly indebted to Matthias Siegmann and Stefanie Stegemann-Boehl.

cases--if there is even a discussion about these problems at all. In such situations, an exchange of experience, by way of comparative law and ethics, is certainly a first important step to an international assimilation, if not unification, of rules of conduct and investigation. For this reason, the initiators of this contribution deserve acknowledgement for providing a forum in which to illuminate misconduct in science from an international perspective.

My own chapter will begin with a systematic survey on various case categories of misconduct in science, including reports on a few cases of misconduct in the Republic of Germany that have become publicly known, and also a speculation about possible reasons for the scarcity of information in this area. In a second section, I will attempt to evaluate the various cases of misconduct of researchers in light of the German law, as compared with the American legal situation. This will lead us to the proposition that the first line of defense against the phenomenon of misconduct in science could be at the level of the individual research institution, by way of self-monitoring of the research community--such as the measures taken by the Deutsche Forschungsgemein-schaft (DFG), a German research foundation (comparable to the National Science Foundation in the United States).

INCIDENTS OF MISCONDUCT IN SCIENCE IN GERMANY

Types of Misconduct

The concept of misconduct is rather broad and, especially at its boundaries, flowing and disputable. For our purpose, however, it may suffice to describe the types of misconduct in a more general way. By doing so, I would like to make use of a classification that is orientated to the various stages in the research process, as it seems already widely accepted in the American discussion of these problems.[3]

On the first level, the *production stage*, we must distinguish among plagiarism, fabrication, and falsification of data. When talking of *plagiarism*, we mean the illegitimate appropriation of another's ideas, data, or analysis. *Fabrication* is the recording of data without having conducted the experiment from which the data is gleaned. *Falsification* is the false recording or altering of observations.

Beyond these "classical" cases of misconduct in the production stage, however, is a group that includes cases in which research groups were intentionally distorted, or substances were experimentally procured by another researcher (although in such instances of destruction it may be odd to speak of "production" as its true counterpart).[4]

The next level, the *reporting stage,* is misrepresentation and nonrepresentation of data, such as the act of "cooking," "trimming," or "shading" data, the failure to cite side effects, and the exaggeration of claims or complaints.

On the third, the *dissimulation stage*, we must distinguish between cases of unacknowledged collaborators on the one hand and so-called honorary authorship on the other. In addition, we should also think of simultaneous submissions of manuscripts to journals, as well as the case (which is close to plagiarism) of a reviewer who "pirates" data in a submitted manuscript. If we take the notion of "misconduct in science" in a broad sense, we could even include cases of failure to acknowledge preprint readers, data sources, anonymous reviewer comments, and funding support. These cases can be considered as a foreground of plagiarism.

Finally, in the *evaluation stage*, misconduct may be seen in the failure to provide raw data for replication; or, of particular importance, in cases where those involved remained silent when there was good reason for suspecting the occurrence of misconduct.

PUBLICLY REPORTED CASES OF ALLEGED MISCONDUCT IN GERMANY

So far, in the Federal Republic of Germany the number of publicly reported cases of alleged misconduct has been rather small. The majority of cases that have been discussed thus far concern misconduct during the production stage. Some of these cases are still rather atypical, when compared with American cases. For example, in the United States, most cases investigated so far have been related to the biosciences; whereas in Germany some of our cases are in the areas of pure science and the humanities.

As an example of a case of plagiarism--which even led to a disciplinary proceeding--I would like to mention the (unnamed) case of a professor of mathematics whose habilitation thesis corresponded heavily to another mathematician's monograph, without expressly quoting the passages taken from the exploited monograph. The professor could not argue the fact that he had mentioned the monograph in his foreword, because he had done so in a manner that seemed to express views that were both different and distant to the original work. In this case, the scientist concerned was deprived of his *venia legendi*, that is, his professorial faculty of lecturing mathematics.[5]

Another case of misconduct that occurred several years ago, but that has just come up again quite recently--with tremendous public attention because of the high reputation of the person charged with plagiarism--is the case of a professor of philosophy, Elisabeth Ströker (who, ironically, had not long before published a collection of papers on "ethics in science").[6] A faculty member charged that large parts of her doctoral dissertation on *Zahl und Raum* (number and space) had been taken from Bertrand Russell and Ernst Cassirer, without expressly giving credit to the original work.[7] This charge has meanwhile been confirmed by the philosophy faculty of Cologne University, where Ströker is presently located. They concluded that, having graded the dissertation, they would not have granted the PhD.[8] Now it is up to the original faculty of Bonn University (where Ströker received her PhD) whether the degree will be revoked; and, if this is the case, whether the next degree of doctor phil. habil., which is normally based on the PhD, also will be revoked. While this proceeding is pending,[9] professor Ströker is continuing to teach--and has even presented at a seminar on "ethics in science."

With regard to fabrication and falsification, I should mention the case of Ernst Rupp, a physicist in Berlin who in the 1920s and 30s published sensational experiments of the interference of electronic rays--which were completely fabricated.[10]

In addition, though already known in the US,[11] I should also mention the cases of Robert Gullis and Hasko Paradies because they serve as good examples for the international dimension of these problems.

The case of the English biochemist Robert Gullis usually is treated as an English case of misconduct in science; however, it is also a German one because this is where the misconduct originated. This young English researcher with excellent prospects had, from 1975 to 1976, worked as scholar in the Max-Planck-Institute for Biochemistry near Munich. Some apparently significant research results in the field of neurotransmitters led to a number of publications by his research group, including papers in *Nature*. Later, after Gullis's return to England, his research group did not have any further progress because the experiments that Gullis pretended to have conducted could not be reproduced. Gullis had to concede that all his experiments were not performed, but instead were invented by him. Consequently, the publications had to be retracted. Yet, whereas Gullis lost his position in England, his coauthors, who had believed in him, remained without any sanction.[12]

More successful than Gullis, at least at the beginning, was the professor of biology Hasko Paradies in Berlin. Based on impressive inquiries on the crystallization of transfer ribonucleic acids, which were published in international journals, he was appointed as professor in 1974. Then, in 1982, an international team of leading biochemists was able to prove that his publications had been fabricated. When the Free University of Berlin instituted an investigation committee, Paradies (in May 1983) agreed to a deal with his employer, which asked for his dismissal; in return, the university promised not to proceed with further investigations into the former "paradise" in professor Paradies' former institute.[13]

Finally, I should mention another, again atypical, case of the molecular biologist E. Wellnikow.[14] In 1984, she had distorted bacterial cultures designed to investigate human sexual appeal substances--an experiment performed by her direct superior and, then, friend. Unlike other cases of misconduct, however, where a scientist will act for egoistic reasons, Ms. Wellnikow came forth because she wanted to prevent the commercial exploitation of ethically doubtful research results by her superior. This case does not seem to have had any personal consequences for her, because her superior stopped his experiments after this "attack," and refrained from any steps against his former girlfriend.

CONFIDENTIALLY TREATED CASES

Considering the rather few publicly discussed cases, it is certainly fair to assume that the number of confidentially treated cases is probably higher. For instance, a student of mine[15] (who is working on the legal implications of misconduct in science in her doctoral dissertation) obtained in personal interviews information that there had been a very clear case of fabrication and falsification of data in one of our leading centers for cancer research. This case was concluded by the termination of employment of the researcher concerned (however, this fact did not prevent him from finding a position in industrial research). There were no other sanctions against the researcher.

Another instance (obtained by my student on confidential basis) is a clear case of abuse of the peer-review system. A reviewer took data from the paper he reviewed and incorporated it into his own database. Even worse is the fact that quite a lot of effort was needed (by the chief of his lab) to convince the misbehaving reviewer to delete the data he had illegally acquired. Once again, there were no disciplinary measures. In general, there seems to be a common assumption among German scientists and scholars that fabrication and falsification of data in German research is, to say the least, not unknown, though the amount and seriousness of it is difficult to quantify. Of particular suspicion in this context are congress abstracts that are not published as originals, which seems to be the case in about 40 percent of all abstracts. Another example of misconduct, which is certainly not uncommon, is that of individuals who remain silent even though misconduct is suspected.

THE LACK OF INFORMATION AND PUBLIC DISCUSSION ON ISSUES OF MISCONDUCT

It is rather easy to explain why we have so few publicly reported cases of misconduct in science in Germany. Indeed, the situation is comparable to that in the US at the end of the 1970s, when the total amount of misconduct cases may have been similar to those of the early 1980s, but misconduct in science was not a public topic. In order to reach the level of public interest seen today, spectacular cases, such as those of Elias Alsabti, Marc Straus, or John Darsee in 1982 had to become known. Since the German incidents are so far not comparable to the American ones, there is a lack of interest on the part of the media and, thus, by the as-yet-unaware public.

As long as there is no public interest in such issues, however, executive and legislative opinion makers are not inclined to give attention to this delicate problem; especially because of the fact that our science and university policy is just now deeply involved in solving the problems posed by the transition of the former socialistic ideologic East German research institutions into a system of freedom of science and research.

Last, but certainly not least, the scientific community is quick to handle problems of misconduct (if recognized at all and not simply ignored) in the most confidential manner as possible. There is a fear that "sleeping dogs may be awakened" if public confidence in the integrity of the academic world is shaken by openly discussing potential misconduct of scientists. Perhaps this is best illustrated by the demands, which have arisen in connection with relevant discussions within the DFG, that a working paper of one of my assistants, dealing with legal implications of misconduct in science, should be qualified and handled as "confidential."

It is quite clear that this "wall of silence" may also cause potential whistleblowers to keep suspicion of misconduct to themselves for fear of reprisals.[16] As is shown by examples in the US, the situation can change very rapidly when some spectacular cases become known, and our present tranquillity may turn out to be the calm before the storm. Therefore, it seems of vital importance to obtain more information on the prevalence of misconduct in German scientific research. Were the few cases reported before only "bad apples" or "the tip of the iceberg"? This is even more difficult to answer in Germany than it is in the US, since so far we do not have any reliable empirical data.[17]

Therefore, we can only make a tendentious assessment. This leads to the assumption that the prevalence of misconduct in Germany probably is lower than in the US. This perhaps surprising conclusion can be explained by analyzing the factors that are responsible for misconduct in the US. If I am correct, the main factors contributing to the occurrence of misconduct in science in the US are the great pressure to publish (according to the maxim of "publish or perish"), as well as increasing numbers of financial ties between scientists and industry, and the increasing size of research programs.[18] Under German non-industrial research conditions, factors such as these appear to play a significantly minor role. Moreover, German research units are mostly state-run or otherwise funded by public means. As a result, the individual researcher is, for the most part, already financially equipped in such a way that he/she is not dependent on constantly raising funds by waving his/her publication list. Another factor may be that, so far, joint ventures between academic research and industry are not as frequent and close as to impede (by profit aspects or contractual limitations and discriminations) a free flow of research results and the exchange of data between individual scientists.

Furthermore, since the size of the average research program in Germany is much smaller than comparable American research programs, it is easier to supervise the various members of the research group.

This, of course, is not to say that we do not have to deal with a significant "gray zone" of misconduct in Germany. When observing the increasing dependance of research on so-called "third funds" (granted by private sponsors), which lead to greater financial interweaving between science and industry--and when realizing the increasing tendency of larger research programs that are even more intense due to the growing cooperation on the European scale--it is even more likely that the climate for misconduct in science will increase rather than decline.

MISCONDUCT IN SCIENCE IN VIEW OF THE GERMAN LAW

Possible Legal Sanctions and Other Consequences

In order to understand the handling of misconduct in science by German law, two points must be made clear from the very outset: First, there is no special legislation or other regulation regarding misconduct in science in Germany at all. Second, this does not mean, however, that we have a complete legal vacuum with regard to misconduct in science, but rather that we must resort to norms and rules--some of which were perhaps developed long ago for other types of illegal activities, but can still be applied to misconduct in science. This cannot be done by a wholesale adaptation of other rules, but by distinguishing certain circumstances and preconditions. In Germany these are as follows:

1. The personal status of the researcher, in terms of the type of employment, is the first important condition to consider. For instance, is he/she a state official (*Beamter*)? In the case of most professors or long-term research personnel at state universities, the scientist is governed by (and perhaps prosecuted according to) the same disciplinary rules as any other state official; if the researcher's work is part of an official function, any misconduct in science may be a culpable violation against the state, as well as the university.[19]

   Depending on the gravity of the violation, the code of ethics--referred to as the *Disziplinarordnung(en)* by the various German states--provides sanctions starting from mere admonitions or reprimands, progressing to fines or salary reductions, and ending with dismissal. This catalogue of sanctions seems somehow comparable to those proposed by the NIH and NSF regulations.

   If the researcher is not a state official, but has instead the status of a private employee, the aforementioned code of ethics does not apply. In this case, only measures provided by the labor law are applicable, starting with less severe admonitions but eventually ending with dismissal.

   If the researcher concerned is a physician, he/she may also face sanctions of the special professional code of ethics, established by the various regional chambers of physicians with approval by the respective State Ministry of Health.[20]

2. The sanctions considered so far primarily depend on the personal status of the researcher concerned; the type of misconduct is of secondary relevance. The type of misconduct becomes more important when we look for

sanctions beyond the personal employment status of the researcher. Without attempting to present a comprehensive report within this chapter, with regard to important types of misconduct, I will give specific examples of possible sanctions and the obstacles connected with them.

Plagiarism does not only occur during the production stage of research, but is also well known in other areas of writing and opinion making. However, the German law does not recognize plagiarism by a special legal definition; instead, plagiarism is commonly described in a more nontechnical sense as "conscious appropriation of foreign intellectual goods."[21] According to the German copyright law, the foreign ideas must have been appropriated for personal purposes, and must already have reached a certain inner and outer form in terms of a "work."[22] Thus, a mere idea, though expressed, is not protected per se. To have the quality of a "work" does not, however, require its publication. So even a research design can be treated as a "work" if it is the expression of a personal intellectual effort by the author. Yet, in order to encourage scientific freedom and free flow of ideas, our federal Supreme Court would not consider a scientific contribution to be protected (even if it is characteristic of a scientific contribution or article) unless it is qualified by a self-creative format, with the intellectual contents--that is, the research result--remaining free.[23] Therefore, it is questionable whether the misconduct by Elias Alsabti, had it occurred in Germany, would have been treated as a violation of copyright law. However, according to the aforementioned requirements, if the plagiarised object is a protected "work," the plagiariser may be punished according to § 106 Urheberrechtsgesetz, with a fine or imprisonment up to three years. Besides this criminal sanction, the wronged author may have a civil claim for restitution, damages, and future omission. But since all these sanctions require proof of intended plagiarism, in practice it is not easy to prove those claims.

If copyright law is not applicable, the wronged author may still have civil claims for violation of his/her so-called "general personal right," comparable to the right of privacy.

3.   Fabrication and falsification of data also are not punishable, as such, in Germany. If a researcher recorded invented or falsified data in his/her lab book, it merely would be a so-called "written lie," which is not punishable as such. However, if afterwards he/she made changes to already-listed data after having lost the free disposition over the lab book, such "doctoring of a lab book" could be punishable according to § 267 StGB (German Penal Code).

4.   If data is destroyed, the criminal sanction for destruction of physical goods (Sachbeschädigung) may be applicable (§§ 303, 303 cStGB), and civil damages may be claimed (§ 823 sect. 1BGB, German Civil Code).

5. If a researcher has acquired a research grant by misrepresentation of data, he/she may be ordered according to civil law to repay the grant. This, however, presupposes that the researcher can be proven to have intentionally misrepresented the data, and to have anticipated that otherwise the sponsor would not have provided the funds.

These requirements are even more crucial with regard to a criminal prosecution. This is particularly true if the money comes from a private sponsor, such as the Deutsche Forschungsgemeinschaft, which, though receiving its money from public funds, distributes it as a private organization according to private law. In this case, a misrepresentation of data could only be handled according to our German provision for fraud (§ 263 StGB), requiring proof that the error was intentionally caused by the misrepresentation, and that there was intentional damage to the sponsor. Since intentional damage to the sponsor is difficult to prove in cases of subsidies (because this money is to be spent in any case), our legislator has made a special provision for fraudulently appropriating subsidies. In these cases, only proof of intentional misrepresentation of data is required, whereas the question of some causal damage to the sponsor remains irrelevant (§ 264 StGB). This provision, however, is only applicable to public research grants, which is only a small portion of German money given to the research community.

If it is not a misrepresentation but merely a nonpresentation of data, as in cases of selective reporting, then at what point can we speak of "misconduct" in legal terms? This borderline is particularly difficult to determine when the researcher is only expected to present a summary of his or her project but not a detailed survey of the results. Such a summary may create a tendency for bias, with researchers arbitrarily leaving off data that does not fit; this type of nonpresentation is, in fact, a case of misrepresentation.

6. In the dissimulation stage, the legal situation is clearer because there are at least some legal rules for authors' practices. With regard to unacknowledged collaboration, our federal and relevant state laws require that in a publication of research results all coworkers who have contributed scientific information must be named as coauthors.[24] This applies not only to written publications, but also to research results made public, such as by mass media. The rationale of these provisions is to allow greater recognition of the achievements of junior researchers. As long as a coworker does not wave these rights, he/she may even have a civil damage claim against his/her superior or other coresearchers. In addition to these rights drawn from university law, a researcher who was "left out" could also invoke copyright law, as long as the publication concerned qualifies as a "work."

With regard to honorary authorship, the situation in Germany is not very much different from that in the US. It is particularly difficult when both the actual and the honorary author consent to inclusion of the honorary author's name--either with the actual author's name, or by itself. The true authors certainly cannot be compelled to agree to naming a senior as coauthor, contrary to the facts. If, on the other hand, someone has been named as coauthor without consent, the other author(s) could be punished for forgery (§ 267 Penal Code) because of falsely presenting someone as author who in fact does not stand behind this statement. In addition, the "author against his will" may also sue for civil damage, restitution, and future omission.

7.   As to the failure to acknowledge preprint readers, data sources, anony-mous reviewer comments, and funding support, we find in German law merely the duty to indicate the true source.[25] But even this duty has a different legal basis, depending on the character of the publication con-cerned: The copyright law can only be invoked if the publication concerned is qualified as a "work," as discussed before. Otherwise, the right to be cited has to be based on the "general personal right" of the author.

8.   In the case of "pirating" data in a submitted manuscript, the same rules as in cases of plagiarism could be applied. This is not easily carried out, however, since the reviewed author can bring charges only after he/she determines the identity of his/her reviewer, which usually is kept secret. To overcome this difficulty we should have a right of disclosure against the journal or the sponsoring organization; so far, this does not exist. The same is true with regard to obtaining access to the abusing reviewer's materials; even if the reviewer's identity has been disclosed, he/she could hardly be forced to open his/her lab book to a suspicious colleague.

9.   The legal situation becomes even weaker when we come to the evaluation stage, as in cases of failure to provide raw data for replication or of remaining silent when the occurrence of misconduct is suspected. Other than having limited control within the employment relationship, no sanc-tions are available.

How Misconduct is Handled in Practice

This survey on possible legal actions, despite certain reservations that had to be made, may have created the impression that the legal instruments already at hand in Germany are sufficient to handle the problem of misconduct in science. This conclusion is wrong. To correct this situation, we must look at how matters of misconduct are handled in practice. To date, I do not know of any case of misconduct in science, in the public or in the private industrial sector, that has been tried before a German criminal court.[26] This could be partly explained by the reluctance of the prosecuting authorities to take these new and rather delicate affairs to task. Another explanation may be that the various parties involved in cases of misconduct would prefer an informal settlement of the conflict in order to prevent a potential public scandal. The case of Hasko Paradies could serve as a good example of this attitude.

Therefore, only administrative proceedings aimed at revoking research subsidies because of abuse by the grantee have become known.[27] A particularly appalling example may be the case of the German chemical factory of Imhausen, which had become known worldwide because of its involvement in the construction of a factory for chemical weapons in Lybian Rabta. Not only did Imhausen commit war-control crimes by illegally exporting supplies, it had even received --though nominally for another project--significant public research grants. Another court case that has become known, but that appears to be pending, was a civil sue against a "whistleblower" for defamation.

On the whole, to date, these already existing state laws and comparable regulations of public character have not begun to have been applied in the core area of misconduct in science.

MISCONDUCT IN SCIENCE AND SELF-CONTROL
BY THE RESEARCH COMMUNITY

The deficiencies at the legal level mentioned above mean that measures against misconduct in science are primarily, though not exclusively, the responsibility of the scientific community as such. Research institutions have the primary responsibility for ensuring that published research results are based on methodologically correct procedures, thus justifying public confidence in these results.

On the other hand, however, research institutions also must ensure that scientific engagements are kept sufficiently free from external interventions, and that the researchers in the future will not be subjected to undue preventative control by state authorities. The challenges of misconduct can be managed only if the research institutions are ready to develop policies against misconduct in science, as has taken place in the US. Initially, this requires the development of a procedural scheme for handling allegations of misconduct, as well as a basic description of what misconduct in science is.

It is also quite clear that this task cannot simply be left to the individual research institutions because their general scientific competence in such matters is, as already evidenced by American instances,[28] no guarantee that misconduct allegations will be treated adequately.

That is why research organizations above the level of individual research institutions, such as the Deutsche Forschungsgemeinschaft, should lead the way in developing guidelines or at least in giving advice as to how to handle cases in misconduct in science. As Robert Rosenzweig put it, "it is far better to have procedures in place with no cases than to have one case and no procedure."[29] It is with this in mind that the DFG is about to develop guidelines for handling allegations of misconduct, as well as descriptions of relevant types of misconduct.

Although so far nothing definite can be said as to which course the DFG is going to take, as Vice-President of the DFG, I would at least venture to guess that guidelines that already have been adopted in other countries, like those of the NSF and the NIH, will certainly be referred to for comparison and eventually as a guidance. However, these guidelines must not be fully adopted, since the German point of view is not identical to the American view. The American models might be modified at least in two aspects: First, more precise definitions for the various cases of misconduct must be determined, although there may still be a need for a general clause; Second, a less formal procedure should be structured to avoid "bureaucratic overkill."[30]

The reservations toward the American example are due primarily to national peculiarities; they should not serve as an impediment to reaching the final goal of efficient management of misconduct in science using legal means on an international scale.

NOTES

1   See the case of the English biochemist Robert Gullis, who used a two-year research stay at the Max-Planck-Institute for Biochemistry near Munich in the years 1975-1976 exclusively for fabricating experiments (for details, see A. Flsing, *Der Mogelfaktor* (Hamburg, Germany: Rasch & Rhring, 1984), 103-7.

2   Publications in foreign scientific journals are found in the Gullis case, as well as in the case of Hasko Paradies. See Flsing, *Der Mogelfaktor*, 21.

3   See, for instance, M.J. Littlejohn and M. Matthews, *CRS Report for Congress, Scientific Misconduct in Academia: Efforts to Address the Issue* (Washington, DC: Library of Congress, 1989), 2.

4   Compare this to the Wellnikow case reported below.

5   His legal suit against this revocation before an administrative court has so far not been successful. See Verwaltungsgericht Arnsberg, in, Verffentlichungen der Umweltminister-Konferenz. Informationen zum Hochschulrecht (Bonn, Germany, 1989), 170; an appeal is still pending.

6   Compare this to *Die Zeit*, 26 October 1990, p. 22.

7   See M. Soreth, *Kritische Untersuchung von Elisabeth Strökers Dissertation ber Zahl und Raum, nebst einem Anhang zu ihrer Habilitationsschrift* (Cologne, Germany: Eigenverlag, 1990). (Soreth, as faculty colleague, had been the "whistleblower" in the Ströker case).

8   See the report in *Klner Stadtanzeiger*, 5 March 1991, p. 10.

9   Contrary to the report cited in *Klner Stadtanzeiger*, Ms. Stegemann found out in a personal interview with Ms. Soreth, the "whistleblower."

10   See Flsing, *Der Mogelfaktor*, 20, 74.

11   See P. Woolf, "Deception in Scientific Research," *Jurimetrics Journal* 29 (Fall 1988):67-95. Woolf classifies the case of Gullis as an American case.

12   For more details to this case, see Flsing, *Der Mogelfaktor*, 103-7.

13   *Ibid.*, 21.

14   Compare this to G. Haaf and B. Hochberg, *Der Erogenfaktor oder wie die deutsche Gelehrtenrepublik ihre Unschuld verlor* (Munich, Germany: Meyster, 1985). As to this case, however, it should be kept in mind that because of the novelistic manner of the report, it is difficult to recognize the borderline between facts and fiction.

15   Stefanie Stegemann-Boehl.

16   The potential consequences of whistleblowing for a colleague of a suspect could be easily demonstrated by the case of Ströker/Soreth: When the latter had publicly accused her colleague Ströker of plagiarism when preparing her dissertation, anonymous fly sheets emerged calling for a "demo in favour of Ms. Ströker" and denouncing the whistleblower as "nut" and "murderer" (of Ströker's honour). See *Klner Stadtanzeiger*, 5 March 1991, p. 10.

17   As to the problems of estimating evidence in the United States, see Woolf, "Deception," 72.

18   See Littlejohn and Matthews, *CRS Report*, 3.

19   As to this situation, see the case of plagiarism in mathematics described above.

20   See, for instance, 54, sect. 2, 57 Kammergesetz Baden-Wrttemberg.

21   K. Vinck, in *Urheberrecht*, 7th ed., ed. F.K. Fromm and W. Nordemann (Stuttgart and Berlin, Germany: Kohlhammer, 1988), 24 and note 1.

22   See 2 sect. 2 Urheberrechtsgesetz (German copyright law).

23   See the survey by H. Hubmann, "Der Schutz wissenschaftlicher Werke und der wissenschaftlichen Leistung durch das Urheberrecht nach der Rechtsprechung des Deutschen Bundesgerichtshofs," in *Urheberrecht und kulturelle Entwicklung, Festschrift zum 60 Geburtstag von Ulrich Uchtenhagen* ed. Schweizerische Vereinigung fr Urheberrecht (Baden-Baden, Germany: Nomos, 1987), 175-87, esp. the (partly critical) summary, 185 and following.

24   See, for example, 58 Universittsgesetz Baden-Wrttemberg.

25   See 63 sect. 1 in connection with 51 Nr. 2 Urheberrechtsgesetz.

26   With regard to a disciplinary proceeding that had been dismissed in the 1950s, see "Dienststrafhof fr die Lnder Niedersachsen und Schleswig-Holstein," in *72 Deutsches Verwaltungsblatt,* ed. C.H. Ule (Cologne, Berlin, Bonn, and Munich, Germany: 1957), 461-64.

27   See the short notice in "Spiegel" 1991, nr. 1, p. 16.

28   See A. Mazur, "The experience of universities in handling allegations of fraud or misconduct in research," in AAAS-ABA National Conference of Lawyers and Scientists, Project on Scientific Fraud and Misconduct, "Report on Workshop Number Two," 1989, 67-93.

29   Cited by W. A. Thomas, "Workshop Summary," in AAAS-ABA, "Report on Workshop Number Two," 1-27, 10.

30   As already warned against by Littlejohn and Matthews, *CRS Report,* 35.

10

The Recombinant DNA Revolution and the Fading of the Concept of "Pure" Science at the Root of Ethical Issues in Biological Research

Vittorio Sgaramella

Research as a means of increasing knowledge should be intrinsically ethical or, at most, ethically neutral. Yet, on the contrary, it has been raising several ethical questions, both thematic and procedural in nature. This trend is becoming acutely evident in essentially all developed countries, mainly in the biomedical sector, due to the potentially rewarding applications of genetic engineering. With genetic engineering, there is a great potential for unethical behavior, such as misrepresentation of data. Therefore, it seems necessary to analyze dispassionately the causes and to discuss ways in which to discourage this trend. Of particular relevance in this context is the need to discourage a utilitarian concept of science and, especially, to decrease the tendency to evaluate the quality of researchers according to the quantity of their publications. This chapter will examine the causes and trends of ethical issues in biological research, with suggestions for avoiding unethical behavior.

The advent of the recombinant DNA technology admittedly has catalyzed a revolution in modern biological research. The most conspicuous developments in this technology interest all the areas of biology: a true "gene rush" has ensued all over the world since the early 1970s, following the discoveries of ligase and restriction enzymes, and the diffusion of gene synthesis, cloning, sequencing, and amplification.

The hopes to exploit both the biosynthetic properties of the gene and its informational content have spurred the proliferation of biotechnology companies and the blossoming of national, regional, and global genome-sequencing programs. Biology has become an important science that is capable of bringing, within close control of the operators, one of the few natural phenomena still largely unbridled--evolution of life. And, accordingly, it is also becoming a "big" science, with its most relevant programs seeing significant budget increases over the last few years.

Illustrious universities are becoming profit-oriented ventures; professors and academic researchers have dual roles as part-time executives and managers; biotechnological companies have replaced academia in setting the trends for fashionable research topics; traditional seminars and reports tend to be substituted by press conferences and releases; and in the university setting, research papers are cleared for publication after extensive reviews, by referees which, unfortunately, are more concerned with patent protection than with scientific value. Research that was once considered "pure" (that is, nongoal oriented) can now become tainted as it contends with fund raising and other commitments. And all of the present-day research, be it pure or less so, is funded and/or committed.

But more relevant to the topic of this book are the ethical issues raised by modern biological research. In my opinion there are two reasons why this research can and must come under the scrutiny of systematic ethical reflection: the first could be called "thematic" and the second one could be considered "procedural."

That scientific research might have thematic issues blurred by ethical ambiguities initially could seem an unlikely hypothesis. After all, research could be viewed as the secular arm of wisdom, the tortuous path leading to the understanding of mankind and the world around him. How could scientific research become unethical? How could the pursuit of truth lead to the accomplishment of evil?

Increase of knowledge has always been synonymous with progress. And I think it still should be. The problem arises when a profound change affects the equation (knowledge equal, or at least leading, to wisdom), turning it into a different equation (knowledge equal or at least leading to power to intervene and to manipulate). For example, a deeper knowledge of the phenomena characterizing development of differentiated cells and their consequent loss of totipotency (that is, the ability of a single cell to generate a fully developed organism according to its potential genetic information), accompanied by a more sophisticated control of the technology of embryo splitting, may lead to the cloning of a superior breed of bovines, and thus of other mammals, all the way up to the primates. This technology is far from being mature, but certainly is within the realm of advanced embryology or, as some refer to it, reproductive engineering. Other ethically ambiguous themes related to genetic engineering (transgenic organisms resulting from gametes, zygotes or embryo manipulations and their environmental release) also could be cited in this regard.

The second reason why research can be unethical is procedural in nature, which includes misrepresentation of data or of programs. This unpleasant phenomenon knows no national boundaries and is probably not dramatically more frequent in the biomedical area than in other scientific quarters, but here it is certainly more serious in light of its effects on health protection. And the impact of the genetic engineering and recombinant DNA revolution on the media--and thus on the public perception of this scientific endeavor--is, in my opinion, devastating, especially in the way it affects the performance of research. It is no wonder that the concept of pure research is becoming blurred. The unwritten code of good scientific practice is losing credibility; the race to obtain huge grants and highly paid consultantships, as well as the exigence of being present in far too many meetings and committees, make it difficult for senior researchers to closely supervise and verify laboratory protocols and results. This leaves younger, less-experienced workers freedom that is not always justified, allowing the infiltration of elements and attitudes that favor unorthodox behaviors.

It is against this background that the specific problem of misrepresentation of data needs to be analysed. According to Goethe, as cited by Max Planck in his 1918 Nobel lecture, "as long as men strive to achieve something, they will always be running into errors." Karl Popper was convinced that "our knowledge grows according to our ability to learn from errors."[1] In James B. Conant's opinion, "science is an adventure, full of errors and guilts as well as of wondrous triumphs: it is an endeavour brought forth by human beings often very fallible and emotional." In his *Teacher in America*,[2] Jacques Barzun recognizes that "science is made by men, with regard to interests, errors and hopes, exactly like poetry, philosophy and the whole human history. To admit this it is not to degrade science . . . on the contrary, it is to appreciate its progresses, which show the genius advancing painstakingly in the mud." And we may conclude this brief and dispassionate apology of errors in science by remembering Max Born, who is credited to have stated that "in science we proceed by trial and error, as we do in a jungle."

All these quotations are excerpted from writings antecedent to the advent of genetic engineering. Since 1970, what Max Born described as a "jungle" because of its epistemological intricacies, is indeed becoming a sociological jungle for its lack of fairness and gentlemanliness. Errors are an intrinsic part of the experimental research activity; mistakes are unfortunately unavoidable, but fraud is intrinsically alien to it. And yet, fraud seems to be occurring more and more frequently. Why is this so?

It has been often and correctly stated that the number of researchers currently active exceeds the total number of researchers that ever existed. It is a fact that several science departments (for instance, genetics) did not even exist in the mid-century universities. Although in most countries the public funding of research has been increased over the past few years, it cannot keep pace with the number of active researchers. As a result, a much fiercer competition for grants exists today. To succeed, scientists must secure highly visible positions and be as conspicuous as possible in the publication sweepstakes. "Publish or perish" is the unfortunate but appropriate motto for this trend--spawning an unwillingness to share data, strains, and cells. The number of scientific journals ready and eager to publish papers is growing fast. In the so-called biotechnology sector, close to forty journals are now available, as compared to zero some twenty years ago. Other sectors in the biomedical area may be experiencing a less-dramatic growth. This proliferation has an explanation: scientific journals can be highly profitable.

With the extreme pressure to publish and the receptivity (or even the stimulatory effect) of so many journals comes a tendency to publish irrelevant, repetitious papers. This deluge of inadequate and useless information submerges those papers that truly deserve publication, circulation, and attention. The publication system becomes clogged and libraries look like busy supermarkets or, indeed, like inextricable jungles. Journals that summarize other journals are becoming more and more popular: scientists find it almost necessary to turn to "News and Views" or "Trends in whatsoever branch" of biological sciences much too frequently, similar to the educated but busy reader preferring to browse through the *New York Review of Books* or *Reader's Digest* rather than read the original texts.

The excess of publications metastasizes the system responsible for the diffusion of scientific results, and exerts a severely negative effect on the progress of science. A recent survey by the Philadelphia-based Institute for Scientific Information has indicated that about 55 percent of the papers published in the widely circulating scientific journals receive no citation whatsoever in the five years following their appearance.[3] In addition, because it is possible to eventually publish anything that loosely resembles a scientific paper, with hastily arranged results or even falsified data, the system is left vulnerable to instances of frequent misrepresentation. The result is one of the most serious threats to the healthy survival of science.

A possible solution, already enacted in some areas, would be to limit the number of publications a researcher can use when applying for grants or position: a rule similar to that used in the tennis or ski world cups, car races, and other sports. In such an instance, only a maximum of, say, ten papers are eligible for use in the researcher's publication list. In time, some of these papers could be replaced with more relevant contributions, as they become available. But the pressure to compile gargantuan lists of titles should eventually be alleviated in favor of better and fewer papers. The review system also could be improved by a diminished number of publications: referees could be induced to do a better job, perhaps with some form of economic compensation--after all, the scientific journals generally make their profits with the aid of the referees. Referees also should be asked to identify themselves in the papers they have declared acceptable for publication.

Another ethical issue related to the procedural aspect is the problem of sharing data,[4] strains, and cells; which, when produced in a publicly funded institution, should be considered as a commonality, as seeds necessary for the propagation of the scientific culture. After all, in the past, plant seeds were considered commonalities. To encourage free circulation of strains and cells, scientific journals might require that authors agree to share such information before accepting their papers for publication.

What can be done to curb the plague of misrepresentation of data? Prevention should be considered first. Usually scientific fraud is committed by young people--mishandlers do not have a long academic life--who generally are disturbed by emotional and behavioral problems.[5] One wonders whether a true effort for preventing the occurrence of such behavior has been contemplated and enacted, in a routine way, as it is done for the prevention of injuries and accidents in the laboratory or clinic. Predictive features are difficult to pinpoint in potential wrongdoers. However, supervisors should pay close attention to researchers with unusual working schedules, who show a marked preference to work by themselves, possibly at night: data fudging is most aptly done under such set of conditions.

A decalogue devoted to unethical behavior in scientific research would be both useful and appropriate for the practicing researcher. Perhaps we should remember some of the values that have allowed our civilization to flourish as it has done since the times of ancient Greece. It is a significant experimental finding that the unit cell of the DNA double helix in its B form perfectly resembles the golden ratio feature on the facade of the Parthenon, crowning the acropolis of Athens since the time of Phidias and Pericles. Such a coincidence should urge us to strive to recover and re-elaborate the underlying ideals of *callos cai agathos*, of beautiful and fair, that should be treasured by everyone (the scholars in particular). At stake is the very survival of science and, through its beautiful and fair practice, of human civilization.

NOTES

1   K.R. Popper, *Congetture e confutazioni* (Bologna: Il Mulino, 1972), 2.
2   J. Barzun, *Teacher in America* (Garden City, NJ: Doubleday-Anchor Books, 1964), 90.
3   D. Hamilton, "Research Papers: Who's Uncited Now?" *Science* (4 January 1991): 25.
4   S.E. Fienberg, M.E. Martin, and M.L. Straf, eds., *Sharing Research Data: A Report of the National Research Council* (Washington, DC: National Academy Press, 1985).
5   A. Kohn, *False Prophets: Fraud and Error in Science and Medicine* (Oxford, England: Blackwell, 1986).

11

Fraud and Misconduct in Medical Research: Causes and Control, a United Kingdom View

Raymond Hoffenberg

A few years ago, spurred no doubt by publicity given to the problem in the US, the editor of the *British Medical Journal*, Dr. Stephen Lock, carried out what he referred to as a "non-systematic survey" to get some idea of the prevalence of misconduct in medical research in Britain.[1] The method he chose was simple; it relied on the smallness of the medical community in the country to ensure that most cases would be known about. He wrote to eighty people, mostly professors of medicine or surgery, or editors of medical journals, asking whether (a) they knew of cases of fraud that had not already been publicized, and (b) a mechanism existed in their medical school or institution for dealing with future cases. Seventy-nine of the eighty responded. Over half of them knew of hitherto-unreported instances of medical misconduct, mostly firsthand. Only three of twenty-nine institutions had mechanisms for investigating misconduct. Most of the cases disclosed by this survey had not been formally investigated, but had been settled --in a curiously British way by an unexplained resignation or unpublicized removal of a degree or membership of an exclusive academic society. In the old days, one presumes, the guilty one would have been sent to "the colonies."

This rather crude but illuminating survey suggested that fraud in medicine in Britain was far more prevalent than had been assumed, that the published instances represented the tip of an iceberg, and that our medical schools had not given much thought to the problem or made preparations to deal with allegations. "The next stop," said Lock, "should be for the British authorities to recognize the situation and resolve to tackle it." Not being one to let grass grow under his feet, he called on the then-president of the Royal College of Physicians of London (now the author of this contribution) to persuade him and his college to do something about it. The outcome, almost two years later, was an official report of the college on "Fraud and Misconduct in Medical Research; Causes, Investigation and Prevention" published in February 1991, which forms the basis of this chapter.[2]

THE PATHOGENESIS OF SCIENTIFIC FRAUD

In our report, we identified the same major pathogenetic factors that had been discussed by Petersdorff,[3] Woolf[4] and others: pressure to publish; personal financial gain; vanity and self-aggrandizement; personality deficiencies or psychiatric illness. Despite the outcome of Lock's survey, the working party that produced the report felt that the scale of medical misconduct in Britain was substantially less than in the US. If this is true and the judgement was purely subjective, there are plausible explanations of the disparity.

Petersdorff pointed out the great intensity of competition in the US: to get into medical school, to win research grants, to move up the academic ladder. Success depends to an inordinate and unjustifiable extent on the number of papers published by the applicant. "Promotion committees count and weigh papers but do not read them."[5] While similar pressures exist in Britain, the intensity of competition is far lower. Petersdorff also drew attention to the extraordinary size of science in the US. Large group projects compete for relatively scarce but bountiful awards. Success depends on productivity, and this creates a self-propelling impulse. Department heads employ large teams to carry out large-scale research, to produce a lot of papers, to attract funds, to employ more people, to conduct yet more research. . . . This circular activity leads to multi-authored papers and, more seriously, to lack of personal supervision.

Woolf has commented that several of the most spectacular frauds have taken place in laboratories where the number of papers published each year significantly exceeds the norm.[6] Science in Britain is smaller; we all know one another; teams are smaller and more intimate; supervision is easier (however, this doesn't guarantee that it is meticulous or always provided). Woolf took a closer look at the provenance of some of medical science's most notorious frauds. In drawing attention to the questionable practice of departmental heads having their names attached as coauthors of all papers emanating from their laboratories, she cited the much tramped-over case of William Summerlin, working at the Sloan-Kettering Institute in a group supervised by Robert A. Good. Over the preceding five years, Good had been the author of 342 papers (an average of 68 per year), 325 of which were coauthored with a total of 136 different scientists. It is quite unreasonable to expect anyone--not even a man of Good's energy and intelligence--to supervise in detail the work of so many people. Peter Medawar, who wrote and thought much about the topic of scientific fraud, argued that most directors assume--and as a rule rightly--that young recruits from good schools and with good references will abide by the accepted and well-understood rules of professional behavior.[7] We must look elsewhere to lay the blame for aberrant conduct.

If a departmental head has not personally supervised or otherwise been actively involved in the work of his laboratory, should he allow his name to be attached as a coauthor? There are many pressures on him to do so. A junior colleague may urge him to lend his prestige to the paper, which would reflect well on the junior; a pharmaceutical company or other sponsor may insist on his participation to add weight to a publication for obvious commercial reasons; by adding his name to all departmental papers, the head and the department become recognized as productive, which sets in train the circle of success I outlined earlier. Success in research departments is often equated with size.

Much has been written about the impact of potential financial rewards as an inducement to our less-scrupulous colleagues to commit scientific fraud. Doctors or medical scientists are not immune from such pressures. As Medawar has said, "Some policemen are venal, some judges take bribes and deliver verdicts accordingly; there are secret diabolists among men in holy orders . . . moreover, some scientists fiddle their results or distort the truth for their own benefit."[8] There seems little to add to his comment, but the topic will be further considered under "Prevention."

The incentive of vanity is also well-recognized--George Santayana said, "the highest form of vanity is love of fame." Recognition of merit by one's scientific peers is greatly prized, leading as it does to invitations to speak at conferences, to give notable lectures, to write guest reviews, as well as to prizes and awards. Medawar believed "the most important incentive to scientific fraud is a passionate belief in the truth and significance of a theory or hypothesis which is disregarded or frankly not believed by the majority of scientists."[9] This being so, an initially well-intentioned scientist may be conduced to fabricate results to persuade his colleagues to accept what to him is a self-evident truth. Lewis Thomas believes "it is an impossibility for a scientist to fake his results and get away with it"--unless the work is so trivial that no one bothers about it.[10] If the work is of real significance, other workers will try to repeat it and the truth will soon emerge. Appreciation of the soundness of this statement raises doubts about the rationality of some of science's miscreants.

WHAT CAN BE DONE TO PREVENT SCIENTIFIC MISCONDUCT?

Steps to prevent misconduct arise naturally from consideration of its causes. It is highly unlikely that it can ever be entirely eliminated; medical scientists will always include among their number a few rotten apples (but then, which profession does not?). The hope is that the generally accepted processes of peer review and the opportunities for verification will expose most instances of fraud, at least deterring misconduct. These constraints will only be effective if the environment and atmosphere of the workplace are right, if research institutions lay down and inculcate the highest ethical standards. Indeed, the importance of such standards needs to be recognized by students at an early stage of their careers. Petersdorff quotes a study showing that 88 percent of four hundred medical students had cheated at least once while they were pre-medicals, the most disturbing feature of which was that there was a continuum from this to cheating in medical school, in clerkships, and in patient care--"the culture in which we train our young promotes cheating."[11] A serious indictment, if true.

To counter this, some medical schools provide students with information not only to enhance their awareness of the seriousness of academic offenses such as cheating in examinations, plagiarism, or fabrication of research, but to emphasize that honesty and integrity and exactitude are critical to scholarship in general. This message needs to be reinforced for those beginning careers in scientific research (as formulated in the guidelines prepared by Harvard Medical School); investigators should accept the need for integrity as part of their social responsibility. It is important to emphasize the ethical position and to avoid the inquisitorial approach.

More specifically, steps should be taken to decrease the importance of long publication lists. The emphasis should be on quality rather than quantity. Genuine scientific reports need to be distinguished from abstracts of conference presentations, reviews, or comments; refereed articles from non-refereed. Selection committees and grant-giving bodies might be encouraged to ask candidates to highlight their most significant papers (say, five to ten), and to elaborate on their reasons for choosing them and the part they personally played in their genesis. Selection or promotion committees should let it be known that excellence in teaching or, in the case of clinicians, in the practice of medicine carries as much weight as publication. It has always struck me as absurd that highly suitable candidates for predominantly clinical posts are rejected because their "publication lists are not long enough." The obligation on medical trainees to "publish or perish" not only encourages fraud, but leads to boring, unimaginative, and repetitive research that tends to give academic medicine a bad name.

Attention should be paid to the guidelines on authorship drafted by the International Committee of Medical Journal Editors (the Vancouver group).[12] Authorship should not be a "gift," but should reflect a significant contribution to the work. Participation solely in the collection of data does not justify authorship. In a recent selection committee I questioned a candidate about a list of twenty-eight coauthors of a paper he had written. They were, I was told, clinicians, each of whom had provided the author (and sole investigator) with one or more patients suffering from the relatively rare clinical condition that was the subject of the investigation. Without a promise of coauthorship he thought they would not have bothered to cooperate, so they allowed their names to be attached to a paper they had not read, the scientific details of which they were unfamiliar, and that they, at some stage, would include in their own lists of publications. Recognition of such a dubious basis for authorship would more properly have been made under "Acknowledgements." Editors could quite reasonably be expected to ask each author to justify coauthorship. If there is more than one author, it should be assumed that each has read the paper, is familiar with and has checked the data, is prepared to defend its contents, and has indicated by signature that these assumptions are correct.

The prospect of direct financial gain for the investigator should always heighten suspicion about the authenticity of a study. A recent US Congressional committee disclosed overt financial interest by some investigators in several therapeutic studies, such as ownership of relevant stock. Committees that review the ethics of research projects should be properly informed of all financial aspects of the work, including the sums payable to the investigators for participation and especially for recruitment of research subjects. Here a special problem may arise through the common practice of payment of a fixed sum to the investigator for each subject recruited ("per capita payment"). Under such arrangements, less scrupulous doctors may take patients off satisfactory medication and place them on the drug under trial in order to augment the number of patients admitted to it; doctors have even been known to "invent" patients to meet their commitments, or to supply false data about the same set of patients to different pharmaceutical companies testing different drugs. Checks can and should be made by such companies on the number of patients recruited by comparing them with the number normally seen by the doctor over an equivalent period of time or by other doctors working in comparable practices.

The system of per capita payment should be looked at more critically as it appears to induce less honest doctors to behave in a fraudulent way. Several have appeared before our General Medical Council for disciplinary action. It would be preferable for a fixed total sum to be negotiated between the doctor and the sponsoring pharmaceutical company for recruitment of what is bilaterally agreed to be a reasonable number of patients, as judged from the known experience of that doctor. A flexible attitude by the company toward minor shortfalls would diminish the pressure on a doctor to comply. This, after all, is the approach grant-giving research bodies use when considering applications for funding of clinical studies.

Heads of departments and senior research workers have a clear responsibility to supervise work being done within their institutions. They can only do this properly if the size of their group is manageable. Large groups or departments should be broken up into smaller units that can be adequately supervised by one individual. This should require personal appraisal of experimental results, including scrutiny of raw data such as computer or automated instrument readings.[13] Regular in-house presentation of results with open and critical (friendly) discussion will diminish opportunities for submission of incorrect or fraudulent data. Raw data should be available for inspection even years after completion of a project; computer-held data should be committed to paper for storage.

THE INVESTIGATION AND MANAGEMENT OF COMPLAINTS

Once an allegation of scientific misconduct has been made, a course of action needs to be defined that will incorporate two important principles: (1) to preserve confidentiality (protecting the identify of the "whistleblower" and the "accused") for as long as possible during the course of the procedure; (2) to conform to "natural justice," hence to proceed carefully and systematically, checking the facts at each stage, and not allowing "judgement" to be made until both sides of the case have been heard by an impartial panel. The Royal College of Physicians has recommended a three-stage procedure as a model for institutional action, but each institution should devise its own system to manage a complaint of misconduct. What is important is that such systems should have been thought of ahead of time, a plan of action should have been outlined in advance so that implementation can proceed rapidly and smoothly.

In the first instance, each institution (medical school, research laboratory, pharmaceutical company) should designate and authorize one person to receive allegations of misconduct. The name of this person should be publicized.

Stage I: Receipt of an Allegation

Upon receiving an allegation, the designated person (R) should invite the person (I) making it to write a detailed statement of the nature of the allegation. The case may be dismissed by R if it is thought to be frivolous or without substance; I should be so informed. Anonymity of both I and the accused (A) should be preserved throughout this stage. It may not be necessary to inform A of the allegation. If R feels that there is substance in the allegation, he should proceed to the next stage.

Stage II: Inquiry

R should impanel not more than three independent scientists of distinction and standing to advise him under conditions of strict confidentiality. At this point it may be necessary to inform A that allegations have been made against him. This information should be in writing and, so far as possible, the identity of I should be undisclosed.

If the panel feels for any reason that further action should not take place, they should inform I and A (if he is already aware of the fact). If, on the other hand, the panel feels that further full investigation is warranted, they should report back to R who will inform the appropriate authority and request the panel to proceed to Stage III.

Stage III: The Investigation

This is a formal process of quasi-judicial form. A "bench" of independent representatives of the university or other institution will hear evidence from both sides, including that of witnesses. Clearly, anonymity is no longer possible, so care must be taken not to transgress laws of defamation. The fact and details of the investigation should be circulated only to those who have a real interest in receiving them, and the procedure adopted by the institution for investigations of this kind must be carefully followed.

If a finding of serious scientific misconduct is confirmed, it will be necessary to inform the employing authority, and whatever national body is responsible for setting standards of professional conduct and for taking disciplinary action when these are transgressed. In Britain, this is the General Medical Council. Where appropriate, grant-giving bodies should be informed, as well as editors of all journals in which the malefactor published articles, especially those known to be fraudulent or of questionable validity. Editors should be asked to publish appropriate notices of retraction.

If the finding is one of scientific error but not misconduct, the matter is best dealt with inside the institution itself. The appropriate ethics committee should be informed. If no misconduct has been demonstrated, steps should be taken to preserve the good reputation of the researcher. If there has been publicity about the matter, an official statement may be issued.

CONCLUSION

One must be careful not to overstate the extent of fraud or misconduct in medical science or to overact to it. The vastness--and the considerable rewards--of scientific activity in medicine makes it inevitable that some misconduct will take place. It should be seen in the context of the extraordinary increase in our knowledge over the past few decades. The good far outweighs the bad. If it were at all possible we should all like to eradicate the bad completely. This is unlikely to be achieved. We can, however, do much to contain it by being aware of the danger, by making it hard to go undetected, but especially by strengthening the ethical framework of research so that fraudulent, misleading, bad, or even sloppy science is frowned upon.

NOTES

1   S. Lock, "Misconduct in Medical Research: Does It Exist in Britain?" *British Medical Journal* 297 (1988):1531-35.

2   *Report of the Royal College of Physicians of London. Fraud and Misconduct in Medical Research: Causes, Investigation and Prevention* (London: Royal College of Physicians of London, 1991).

3   R.G. Petersdorff, "The Pathogenesis of Fraud in Medical Science," *Annals of Internal Medicine* 104 (1986):252-54.

4   P.K. Woolf, "Pressure to Publish and Fraud in Science," *Annals of Internal Medicine* 104 (1986):254-56.

5   Petersdorff, "The Pathogenesis."

6   Woolf, "Pressure to Publish."

7   P. Medawar, "The Strange Case of the Spotted Mice," in *The Threat and the Glory* (Oxford: Oxford University Press, 1990), 71-82.

8   P. Medawar, "Scientific Fraud," in *The Threat and the Glory* (Oxford: Oxford University Press, 1990), 64-70.

9   Medawar, "Scientific Fraud."

10 L. Thomas, "Falsity and Failure," in *Late Night Thoughts on Listening to Mahler's Ninth Symphony* (New York: Viking Press, 1983), 108-13.

11 Petersdorff, "The Pathogenesis."

12 E.J. Huth, "Guidelines on Authorship of Medical Papers," *Annals of Internal Medicine* 104 (1986):269-74; International Committee of Medical Journal Editors, "Guidelines on Authorship," *British Medical Journal* 291 (1985):722.

13 Thomas, "Falsity and Failure.

Part II

Conflict of Interest

12

Science, Scientific Motivation, and Conflict of Interest in Research

Roger J. Porter

The search for truth is the most precious fundamental of the scientific process. To denote "scientific veracity" is, to most scientists at least, tautological. Yet scientists, recently exposed as possessing human frailties after all, are under increasing pressure to defend their actions and their image, both from Congress and from the press.[1]

The origin of this pressure is multifactorial. Big science and big-science budgets enhance the likelihood of abuse in the system, as more and more people participate in the process. The history of biomedical science--and especially of the biggest United States funding agency, the National Institutes of Health--has been one of relatively pristine reputations, capturing the public imagination as an institution of dedicated scientists working long hours at low pay to cure human diseases and afflictions. Such a reputation, especially if long-persisting, is an invitation to those whose livelihood depends on exposing scandal in the previously undefiled. Finally, science--most especially biomedical science--is now progressing rapidly. Many biomedical scientists suddenly perceive, for the first time, opportunities for personal gain. That some of these scientists become wealthy has eroded the public image described above, increasing the vulnerability of publicly funded institutions and subjecting individual investigators to scrutiny at a new and intense level. Individual scientists are injured, the community of scientists is fractured, funding sources are endangered, and the public is confused.

So what is really happening? Is science really changing? Are modern scientists really different? How do we reverse this unpleasant decrement in public esteem, which threatens support of the scientific enterprise and promises an overwhelming bureaucracy to micromanage that which remains? This chapter will begin with an analysis of what science is, progress to the nature of the motivations of the investigators who conduct this science, and finally address some aspects of conflicts of interest in research, a dominant and vexing problem for the truth-seeking process we all revere.

THE NATURE OF SCIENCE

The definitions of science (and there are many) have been well summarized by Merton in 1942:

> Science is a deceptively inclusive word which refers to a variety of distinct though interrelated items. It is commonly used to denote (1) a set of characteristic methods by means of which knowledge is certified; (2) a stock of accumulated knowledge stemming from the application of these methods; (3) a set of cultural values and mores governing the activities termed scientific; or (4) any combination of the foregoing.

Clearly, science is a complex entity that is difficult to define, and its perception by the lay community is heterogeneous. But is the new scrutiny on scientists related to science or to the scientists who perform it? To answer this question, let us turn again to Merton for assistance with what he terms the ethos of science, with its four major "institutional imperatives."[2] For the remainder of this chapter I will use the word "science" to be synonymous with the second of Merton's definitions; in this way, I will emphasize the "accumulated knowledge" rather than the process of the persons involved.

1. Universalism

"Universalism" is the first of Merton's institutional imperatives of the ethos of science. It is, more or less, synonymous with "objective," in the sense that science is bound by external validation--such as being consistent with previous observations and knowledge--and is independent of socially determined values such as race or status. When Merton (an American) described this element in 1942, the moment was one of racial and religious exclusion in Europe; Merton's reply, for science, was that "the chauvinist may expunge the names of alien scientists from historical textbooks but their formulations remain indispensable to science and technology. However *echt-deutsch* or 100 percent American the final increment, some aliens are accessories before the fact in every new scientific venture."

The application of the concept of universalism to conflict of interest in the 1990s is just as logical as it was to racism in the 1940s. Although influences external to science can alter the priorities of investigation or the rapidity of progress, the verities themselves are independent of such social pressures. Conflict of interest in biomedical research, therefore, will not alter the eventual outcome of the scientific endeavor. This is not to say that the speed of accomplishment cannot be altered by political forces or by availability of funding. On the contrary, deliberate political emphasis on improved health drives the budget of the National Institutes of Health (NIH), one of the nation's largest research and development efforts. But science is the inexorable extension of "certified knowledge," as Merton puts it, and remains independent of these social factors. This explains, for example, the willingness of the NIH to fund high-quality grant applications from foreign countries, in spite of insufficient funding for many American scientists who apply and wish to receive money for their research. The best science, quite simply, is performed by those scientists who are the most advanced, both intellectually and technologically.

Conflict of interest in research, then, is merely one more social factor that may, either by its direct effect or by the controlling bureaucracy it engenders, alter scientific priorities or the rate of scientific progress; it cannot alter the ultimate outcome, which is truth-dependent and not socially determined.

2. Communism

"Communism" is Merton's term for the communal ownership of scientific information. He notes "an eponymous law or theory does not enter into the exclusive possession of the discoverer and his heirs, nor do the mores bestow upon them special rights of use and disposition." Quite clearly, "scientific advance involves the collaboration of past and present generations."[3] Merton recognized the conflict between the desire for "advancing the boundaries of knowledge"--largely driven by "the incentive of recognition," and the desire for personal pecuniary gain through patents and royalties. That patents would become an accepted--even expected modus operandi for scientists in the 1990s--was not considered. Further, patents imply some degree of secrecy in the development of scientific ideas, delaying entry of the new information in the common body of knowledge.

But secrecy, in all its various forms, does not alter the truth. The process of science moves inexorably forward. Although personal gain may motivate scientists and alter their behavior toward scientific information and the speed with which they disseminate it, and although the emergence of the truth may be delayed, the eventual understanding of nature is unaltered.

3. Disinterestedness

By "disinterestedness," Merton notes the "virtual absence of fraud in the annals of science," based fundamentally on the eschewing of personal gain by the investigator. The mores of science are institutionally derived, and "it is in the interest of scientists to conform on pain of sanctions and, insofar as the norm has been internalized, on pain of psychological conflict." The scrutiny of a scientist's work by colleagues creates a "rigorous policing, to a degree perhaps unparalleled in any other field of activity."[4]

With regard to the relationship between disinterestedness and conflict of interest, little needs to be said. Although half a century has passed since Merton's paper, and fraud is unfortunately no longer exceedingly rare, the fundamentals of science remain undisturbed. It is the emergence of the truth in science, in fact, that is the ultimate exposure, both of fraud and of the defective results, which may emerge from science tainted by conflict of interest.

4. Organized Skepticism

Merton's final imperative of science is "organized skepticism," which is "interrelated with the other elements of the scientific ethos," and is a mandate for the scientist to be prepared to challenge old notions and concepts--even laws --for a new order, should such be required to properly interpret the results of the rational investigations we call science. "The scientific investigator does not preserve the cleavage between the sacred and the profane, between that which requires uncritical respect and that which can be objectively analyzed."[5]

Does conflict of interest in research relate to this imperative of science? It does but, once again, only to document that progress in science is independent, in the long run, of the behavior of scientists. The truth itself is unaffected by cultural perceptions or events. Scientists, in the process of scientific investigations, may occasionally be misled, may--for a time--mislead others, may promise more than can be delivered, and may temporarily confuse both the active scientific participant and the passive observer. In spite of these events, and although the truth comes in fits and starts, the knowledge derived from science inexorably emerges. Those who, for whatever reason, are unable or unwilling to be skeptical of the old, will on some occasions be correct, but on others will be left behind.

We are left, then, as we reflect on the nature of science, with the observation that science itself is independent of the desires of the investigator, and that certified knowledge will, in the end, prevail. The uncontrolled variable we seek, in this inquiry into conflict of interest, is not science, but scientists. The question is, considering that "the truth will out," whether we should be concerned about temporary detours caused by scientists and their conflicts? Are these occasional deviations of any importance? To answer these questions, let us turn from our analysis of science to an analysis of the motivations of the investigators who conduct it.

THE NATURE OF SCIENTIFIC INVESTIGATORS

If scientists, and not science, are the variables on which social phenomena such as conflict of interest hinge, we must then consider what makes scientists want to be scientists and to conduct scientific investigations. For only if we understand the motivations of scientists can we uncover their conflicts. I have previously delineated the four fundamental motivating factors of scientists in a more expanded form, and will summarize here certain concepts from that effort.[6]

CURIOSITY

The most basic of truth-seeking motivations is curiosity. The unadulterated desire to know about human beings and their universe is, in many ways, the foundation of all academia-encompassing disciplines, from science to philosophy, engineering, and sociology. The creation of new thoughts or new knowledge, along with the conveyance of this knowledge (and its foundation) to students, is what drives institutions of advanced education. Scientists may have a specific, limited view of the nature of truth, as it is pursued in the laboratory, but curiosity is the first motivating force.

Curiosity is also the purest of the motivating forces. Inherent in the desire to know is the desire to know the truth. Curiosity is therefore not subject to issues such as conflict of interest or fraud; it is inherently pure; though, in a sense, self-interest is served by the pursuit of the truth.

ALTRUISM

Another fundamental motivating factor, especially in biomedical sciences, is the desire to help the afflicted. In biomedicine, the recently increased opportunity (even for the basic investigator) to observe, in one's own research, the potential for contributing to wellness now makes the field more cohesive than ever. The trail from the laboratory to the clinic is shorter than ever; everyone participates in the thrill of contributing to the development of new, effective therapies.

On the other hand, some have challenged whether altruism really exists. Is not everyone ultimately self-serving, even those who live a life of deprivation in the service to others? The question is worth raising, but cannot be answered; it is an untestable hypothesis.

Does altruism have the potential for engendering bias in research? The desire to "do good" may indeed overwhelm the search for the truth. The intensity of wanting to find a cure for a disease might color the investigator's efforts and temporarily derail the truth-seeking process in the name of "helping people." Sorting out this source of bias from bias incurred in the search for fame (see below) is impossible. In general, however, one considers altruism a minimally biasing motivator of scientific investigators.

FAME

The discussion thus far has dwelt primarily on non-biasing factors that motivate scientists, those in which personal gain is limited and the potential for interfering with the truth-seeking process is minimal. We now move to those motivating factors that have a much greater potential for introducing bias into research--the search for fame and fortune. The first to be considered is the search for fame.

Scientists wish, almost uniformly, to be recognized for their accomplishments. Even the scientific poster in the poorly-lit rear of a display at a scientific meeting is a search for recognition. A continuum of recognition--which is actually a form of academic currency--begins with the obscure poster, moves to a platform discussion, then a plenary symposium, then an invited lecture, a named lecture (sometimes with a prize), all the way to the Nobel Prize itself. All these forms of recognition are strongly reinforcing to the scientist, and provide an impetus to investigate both fully and accurately. The desire for recognition is a major force driving scientific accomplishment.

But the biasing potential of the desire for fame is not negligible, in large part because studies that are "negative" are neither as inherently useful nor as personally rewarding as studies which are "positive." When a scientist makes a prediction and then designs an experiment to test that prediction, the result is almost always more meaningful if the prediction is proved correct. Scientists at all levels, therefore, are desirous of "positive" studies. The graduate student needs them for the doctoral thesis and the most senior scientist needs them in the chase for the Nobel prize. This "push" of the scientific process is external to the truth-seeking effort and can cause the entry of bias; a study may appear to be positive when, in fact, a better study (with less bias) that asks the same question proves to be negative.

One might ask why bias always seems to push the study in a positive direction. If one is not convinced by the reasons above, then imagine a clinical trial of a new drug. Which of the parties involved with the drug wants to see it succeed? The answer is everyone: the patient, the patient's relatives, the nurses, the technicians, the doctors, the funding agency, and the drug company that owns it. Poorly designed investigations, therefore, are much more likely to yield positive than negative results.[7] Indeed, in a cynical sense, the way to prove that a therapy is effective is to test it in a poorly-designed study! A more complete discussion of bias in research is available.[8]

How is the motivation of fame related to the desire for power? Certainly the best U.S. scientists tend to accumulate larger and larger laboratories with "empires" that, at least in part, reflect the scientific prowess of their leader. Does scientific fame lead to power outside the scientific arena? The answer is clearly complex and highly variable. Fame in science does occasionally lead to fortune, which is the next motivating factor to be considered.

FORTUNE

Although society tolerates fame as a reward for scientific achievement--in spite of its biasing potential--society is wary of the accumulation of wealth from scientific accomplishments. Indeed, the same arguments for the need for "positive" studies (described above in the section on fame) apply to the search for fortune. If someone stands to gain monetarily from the outcome of a study, the danger of bias must not be underestimated. This form of bias usually favors positive studies. Only in particularly diabolical settings (for example, company A hires a "scientist" to prove that Company B's therapy is ineffective) is the bias toward a negative study. In general, company-sponsored studies are more likely to be positive than studies funded by a neutral source.[9]

Pecuniary gains come in a variety of forms: direct payments, consultant-ships, gifts, meeting expenses, honoraria, royalties, and equity cover most of the possibilities. The importance of each of these in the bias of scientific studies varies; a full review is available.[10]

The discussion has, thus far, relieved science of culpability in issues of conflict of interest, laid the blame on the doorstep of scientists, and investigated the nature of motivators of scientists, which might cause bias in research. Now we shall address conflict of interest directly, finishing with some notions of how it might be controlled.

CONFLICT OF INTEREST

Conflict of interest is most easily understood by first returning to the motivating forces of scientists and dividing these forces into two groups--those that are truth-seeking and those that are related to personal gain. Assuming that curiosity and altruism are truth-seeking, and that fame and fortune are motivators for personal gain, then the scientist may have multiple "masters" to serve in creating and executing an experiment. If, for example, the scientist is motivated by curiosity and the desire for recognition, then these two masters may (at one time or another) come into conflict. It may not be possible to adequately serve both masters--as was noted by Luke 16:13. Conflict of interest is therefore fundamentally bad, as one master must usually lose. If pecuniary gain is one of the masters, society becomes concerned that monetary gain may inappropriately prevail over purer forms of the truth-seeking process.

CONFLICT OF COMMITMENT

Conflict of interest must be differentiated from conflict of commitment. An excellent summary of the major academic commitments for faculty members has been provided:[11]

1. Assure that research, teaching, and public service obligations to the academic institution are fully met.
2. Abide by restrictions on the type and amount of outside activity, as determined by the academic institution or by subsequent agreements between faculty and the university or hospital administration.
3. Abide by commitments of effort, as specified in contractual research agreements and grant applications.

FRAUD

Conflict of interest is not fraud. When fraud occurs, the tension between the master that dictates truth-seeking and the master which demands personal gain has disappeared; personal gain has become the sole master. Misconduct and fraud are the willful deviation from the truth-seeking process, and although a continuum can occasionally be observed between fraud and conflict of interest, most cases are relatively easily categorized into one or the other.

CONTROLLING CONFLICT OF INTEREST IN RESEARCH

The process of controlling conflict of interest in research is inextricably bound up with the scientific process, the desire for rapid scientific advances, and the issue of competitiveness.

The most difficult question is how to exert some reasonable controls to assure that (a) public funds are well spent and (b) the public at large is not injured by the temporary scientific errors arising from such conflicts.

For university-based science, the first duty for the institution itself is to formulate a reasonable plan for the faculty. It is not possible to improve on the suggestions of the AAMC:[12]

> Develop and disseminate policies that clearly articulate the institution's position on (1) sponsored research, (2) acceptable types and levels of outside financial and professional interests, (3) the need to recognize and deal openly with real or apparent conflicts, and (4) the relationship of faculty and staff to outside institutions and third parties,
>
> Develop procedures for full disclosure to the institution, and to the interested public, of financial and professional interests that may influence, or may be perceived to influence, research activity or other scholarly responsibilities,
>
> Implement enforcement procedures, including appropriate sanctions and notification of university and other officials as required, when apparent violations of institutional rules of federal, state, or local laws occur,
>
> Develop procedures to assure that all research proposals are responsibly prepared and appropriately reviewed in accordance with institutional requirements,
>
> Implement accounting procedures which assure that research funds are expended for the purposes for which they have been provided and that all expected services have been performed.
>
> Assure appropriate and effective management and/or resolution of conflicts of interest through the institutional administrative officers and review committees,
>
> Respond expeditiously and with clarity to questions raised concerning potential conflict situations, and

Serve as a model for faculty behavior and preclude inadvertently exposing faculty to conflicts and concomitant liabilities by avoiding conflicts at an institutional level.

The fundamental integrity of scientists, of course, is the single most important bulwark against bias in research. Since the vast majority of scientists are vigilant against motivations that might distort the truth, many of the institutional suggestions above will prove superfluous. In light of public sensitivity on the issue of fraud and conflict of interest, however, some institutional bureaucracy is required, if for no other reason than to attempt to circumvent federal legislation and all its attendant unpleasantness.

Given all these guidelines to monitor and control conflict of interest, then, where should the emphasis be placed for minimum impact on the scientific process but maximum impact on societal protection? If one first assumes that the monitoring of fundamental laboratory research is, in general, technically difficult and financially impractical, an important first step has been made to delimit the scope and intensity of the regulatory process. That such an assumption is warranted is supported by the observation that society is rarely injured (in any major way, at least) by errors in the basic laboratory. The self-correcting process of science will ferret out errors of any magnitude before these attain public consumption. Since most biomedical investigators are fundamental scientists, the minimization of regulation in this arena is a major step toward "holding the line" on the regulatory process.

So at what point in the scientific process might the public be injured? It is in the late clinical/evaluative phases of testing that bias control becomes critical. Clinical studies are often difficult and expensive to replicate; the usual self-correcting process of science is thereby partly thwarted. Worse, these studies are the final step before mass-marketing to patients who generally have no insight into either the development process or the specific data that support approval of a new drug or device. The public is at the mercy of the veracity of the investigator and the vigilance of the regulatory process. This is not in any way to imply that investigator bias is inherently more destructive to clinical science than to basic investigation; such is certainly not the case. But the potential societal impact of bias in definitive clinical trials is clearly greater than that of basic research. Therefore, if the regulatory process must be energized, logic suggests it focus those energies on clinical/evaluative scientists rather than on fundamental investigators. Further discussion of the advantages and disadvantages of this approach has been considered.[13]

SUMMARY

Conflict of interest in research is a function of scientists and their motivations, not the science they produce. Although scientific priorities can alter the pace of research, the truths derived from the scientific process are relatively free from cultural influences. Conflicts of interest in research may temporarily distort the accuracy of scientific findings, but the truth eventually prevails. Only in certain societally sensitive arenas, such as definitive clinical trials, are vigorous regulations warranted.

The opinions and assertions contained herein are the private views of the author, and are not to be construed as official or necessarily reflecting the views of the National Institutes of Health, the United States Public Health Service, the Department of Health and Human Services, the Uniformed Services University of the Health Sciences, the Department of the Navy or the Naval Service at large, or the Department of Defense.

NOTES

1   US Congress. *Report 101-688 of the House Committee on Government Operations* (1990); J. Henderson, "When Scientists Fake It," *American Way* (March 1990):56-101.
2   R.K. Merton, "Science and Technology in a Democratic Order," *Journal of Legal and Political Sociology* 1 (1942):115-126.
3   Merton, "Science and Technology."
4   *Ibid.*
5   *Ibid.*
6   R.J. Porter and T.E. Malone, *Biomedical Research: The Industry and the Academic Medical Center* (Baltimore, MD: Johns Hopkins Press, in press).
7   T.C. Chalmers, P. Celano, H.S. Sacks, and H. Smith, "Bias in Treatment Assignment in Controlled Clinical Trials," *New England Journal of Medicine* (1983):1358-61.
8   Porter and Malone, *Biomedical Research*.
9   R.A. Davidson, "Source Funding and Outcome of Clinical Trials," *Journal of General Internal Medicine* 1 (1986):155-58.
10 Porter and Malone, *Biomedical Research*.
11 Association of American Medical Colleges. Guidelines for Dealing with Faculty Conflicts of Commitment and Conflicts of Interest in Research. (Washington, DC, 1990).
12 *Ibid.*
3   Porter and Malone, *Biomedical Research*.

13

Conflict of Interest:
A University Perspective

David Korn

The remarkable pace of advancement in the biomedical sciences in the last two decades has truly spawned a revolution. The capacity of the contemporary biomedical investigator to ask penetrating, mechanistic questions, couched in fundamental genetic and molecular language, has led to a breathtakingly rapid convergence of the frontiers of biomedical research, with central issues of human physiology and pathology. No longer must the cutting edge of science involve only primitive model organisms of uncertain relevance to higher life forms, or to man. In remarkable contrast to the state of affairs only twenty years ago, it is now possible for the biomedical investigator to attack directly, in patients and with human tissue samples, some of the most fundamental and intimate details of normal and abnormal cell growth and development. We are privileged to live in a time when powerful new concepts and tools permit us to illuminate some of the most profound mysteries of life.

One consequence of these scientific achievements is that much of the work of the basic biomedical scientist, or of the academic clinical investigator, is perceived as highly relevant to the human condition, with relatively near-term, if not immediate, clinical applicability. Accordingly, interest in and opportunities for the rapid commercial development of the freshest results from even the most fundamental scientific studies have soared. This perception of commercial applicability to problems of human health and disease of high public concern, coupled with the explicit spur of federal government policy (which has over the past decade repeatedly exhorted the biomedical research community to facilitate knowledge and technology transfer), has had a dramatic impact on some fundamental aspects of the culture and behavior of academic medicine. As a result, it has brought to sharp focus a welter of concerns with issues of conflict of interest and conflict of commitment.

Although such intense concern with these matters is of relatively recent vintage within academic medical centers, issues relating to the commercialization of academic research are certainly not new. Indeed, our research-intensive academic institutions have had long experience with them in such fields as chemistry, physics, and the several engineering disciplines. Yet, the interface between the world of academe and the world of commerce is a sensitive one, both complex and potentially problematic. To manage interactions at that interface, institutions have developed specific policies and procedures on consulting and conflict to guide faculty behavior. Under the usually gentle constraints of such policies, transfer of knowledge and technology has been successfully facilitated in support of national economic objectives and to the general benefit of society.

Accordingly, the recent flowering of opportunity for academic-commercial interaction in biomedicine may not seem in itself to be a qualitatively new development demanding of special attention or new policies of oversight and regulation. Yet, there are legitimate and important differences with regard to such commercial entanglements in the biomedical sciences that I believe do raise unique problems that require special attention. In the past few years, the public focus on these issues has been dominated by the interest of a few powerful United States Congressmen, who were initially attracted to the topic of scientific misconduct and have since turned their attention to conflict of interest; in these issues, they have found rich grist for their respective political mills.

This history of Congressional concern has provided an unusual intensity of public attention to these matters; but regrettably, it has shaped the public debate in a way that has blurred important distinctions between the issues of conflict of interest and those of scientific misconduct. It has also tended to define problems and propose remedies in the polarizing context of what has been termed "a clash of two cultures"--the scientific culture and the legal culture.[1] Such a contextual definition is both inadequate and inaccurate. It ignores the fact that most of the activity under examination takes place in academic institutions; and it is the culture of the research university that provides the frame which must ultimately shape the definition of problems and validate proposed solutions.

To begin, it would be well to have some common definition of what is meant by the terms "conflict of interest" and "conflict of commitment." With respect to conflict of interest, one might accept the following useful definition: "A potential or actual conflict of interest exists when legal obligations or widely recognized professional norms are likely to be compromised by a person's other interests, particularly if those interests are not disclosed."[2] Thus, conflict of interest in biomedicine refers to situations in which financial or other personal considerations may compromise, or have the appearance of compromising, a physician's professional judgement in delivering patient care, or an investigator's professional judgement in conducting or reporting research.[3]

The term conflict of commitment, on the other hand, generally refers to an individual's distribution of effort between primary professional obligations of one or another kind and commitments made to what are considered "outside activities." Such activities might, of course, embrace a very broad array, and the term is not meant to imply that such outside activities need be individually, in and of themselves, in any way inappropriate or ill-advised.[4]

Commentators from another university recently put the distinction between conflict of interest and conflict of commitment rather nicely, in the following language.[5] "Conflict . . . has two distinct components--conflict of interest, which most often involves money, and conflict of commitment, which most often involves time. Conflict of interest exists whenever an individual's personal ties could unduly influence a professional judgement. Conflict of commitment exists when an individual's primary loyalties are in doubt." The speakers then went on to opine that "both types of conflict are part of the territory when a university invites the spirit of entrepreneurialism into its midst. Universities are institutions that purport to serve the public good, while entrepreneurs . . . are interested in private gain."

It is important to recognize that the vast majority of basic biomedical research in the United States is conducted in academic settings and is the product of a unique relationship between the federal government and academe. The broad terms of that relationship are straightforward: The government provides major financial support for education and research, while the universities educate scientists and produce knowledge. Under this arrangement, which has been described aptly as a program of investment and not of procurement, the relationship has flourished within an academic environment in which the ultimate responsibility for the conduct of science has rested with scientists, and the maintenance of scientific integrity has depended largely on self-regulation.

At Stanford University, that environment is defined by only a few key policies, enacted by the faculty, that govern the conduct of research and the behavior of research scientists on our campus.[6] The first of these is a Statement on Academic Freedom, the gist of which is captured in a section of its preamble: "Stanford University's central functions of teaching, learning, research and scholarship depend upon an atmosphere in which freedom of inquiry, thought, expression, publication and peaceable assembly are given the fullest protection." A second policy prohibits the performance of any classified research on the campus, as well as any other research that cannot be fully disclosed and published in the open literature.

A third policy is contained in a Statement of Principles Concerning Research, which states in part:

> The transmission of knowledge and conduct of scholarly inquiry are central and complementary functions of the University. They can be carried out

effectively only if scholars are guaranteed certain freedoms and accept corresponding responsibilities. . . . The individual scholar should be free to select the subject matter of his research, to seek support from any source for his work, and to form his own findings and conclusions. These findings and conclusions should be available for scrutiny and criticism, as required by the University's policies on secrecy in research. . . . The above principles circumscribe the University's role with respect to . . . research. They in no way diminish, and indeed they reinforce, the individual researcher's personal responsibility to assure that the sources of funding for his research, and its perceived applications, are consistent with his own judgment and conscience.

In the brevity and substance of these few documents, there is captured for me the very essence of the culture of the research university.[7] Thus, the sparseness of the policies and their near absolute dependence on individual integrity and conscience reflect the fact that the research university constitutes a unique and remarkably complex, but fragile, form of social organization, in which authority is highly decentralized, power widely dispersed, proscription extraordinarily difficult, and prescription invariably suspect.

At Stanford University, from its inception, there has been a concern with matters practical as well as theoretical, and a strong commitment to apply the fruits of scholarly inquiry to the benefit of mankind. University policies and guidelines that address professional interactions between university faculty and the world of commerce are articulated in similarly sparse language that addresses the topics of "conflict of interest" and of "consulting." With respect to conflict of interest, the policy states:

> Most major universities, including Stanford, have taken the position that [consulting relationships] are on balance overwhelmingly beneficial, and there is no disposition to change that view. At the same time, it would be foolish to ignore the fact that some of the complications arising from this state of affairs can cause damage to the University and to the individual, as well. Chief among these complications is that tangled and thorny set of problems embraced by the general title of "conflict of interest."
>
> The issues subsumed under that heading are primarily ethical and as such they are not readily codified to rules of behavior. In any event, this university has never found it necessary to spell out rules or codes of ethics for its faculty and staff. The relationship between the University and its staff assumes that full-time staff members owe their primary professional allegiance to the University and that they will be alert to the possibility that outside obligations, financial interests, or employment can affect the objectivity of their decisions as members of the University community. If those assumptions are valid, as we believe them to be, then no codes or monitoring devices are needed; if they are not valid, then none will suffice.[8]

With respect to consulting, University policy states: "The opportunity for members of the Academic Council to engage in consulting activities outside the University is a privilege long recognized as beneficial both to the individual faculty member and to Stanford. Limits on these activities must be recognized and accepted, however, in order that academic objectives can be insured and the corpus of the University protected."[9] At Stanford that limit is set by restricting consulting activities to one day each week.

Stanford's policy on consulting is clearly permissive, even encouraging, and it served Stanford well, particularly during the decades immediately following World War II, when the flowering of physical and engineering sciences on the campus was accompanied by the remarkable commercial application that gave birth to the "Silicon Valley." That history, in fact, is often cited as one of the premiere examples of successful university-commercial interaction, leading to facilitated transfer of knowledge and technology to the clear benefit of society.

It was against this background and history that the "revolution in biology" erupted on the Stanford campus in the early 1970s and proceeded to transform in fundamental ways the culture of the school of medicine. The school had been translocated to the campus only about a dozen years earlier in the express hope that an institution primarily known for its programs of clinical education and training might be transformed into a center of biomedical research excellence. The relocation of the school was accompanied by some profound changes in the structure and expectations of the faculty: the school adopted a strict full-time system of faculty employment, as well as policies that severely limited the loci of clinical practice of physician faculty members and imposed a pay plan by which all clinical earnings were billed, collected, and administered by a central administrative entity of the school. It is relevant to note that this set of restrictions on medical practice by the faculty was acknowledged to constitute an explicit exception to the university's consulting policy; and it was imposed quite deliberately to promote clinical scholarship and teaching.

During the 1970s, scientific advancements in molecular genetics and immunology flourished in the school of medicine, and arrangements between members of the medical school faculty and diverse commercial enterprises, including a plethora of start-up companies, became increasingly prevalent. These events raised concerns that led to the appointment in 1982-1983 of a select committee to conduct a fresh review and recommend policy on outside consulting activities by faculty in the school of medicine.

The committee report endorsed the existing university guidelines on consulting; but it went on to state,

The Committee recognizes that the scale and extent of non-clinical consulting activities in a number of areas of the life sciences have increased dramatically. It is also quite evident that recent developments in biomedical research made largely in university laboratories have exceptional and unique potential for application to the diagnosis and treatment of human disease. It is important, therefore, that faculty be especially aware that certain abuses of faculty consulting privileges could diminish public trust in biomedical research, in its practitioners and in its applications. Therefore, faculty should be responsive to potential conflicts of interest and of commitment in their consulting activities.[10]

The report then proceeded to the following discussion: "Less blatant, but no less serious to the intellectual aims of the School, are activities which create conflicts of commitment, that is, situations in which the time and creative energy that faculty members devote to consulting is so diversionary as to compromise their commitment to University responsibilities and expectations." To deal with these several concerns, the committee recommended, and the medical school adopted, a formal policy of mandatory disclosure requiring that each member of the faculty report annually to the department chairperson on the nature and scope of nonclinical consulting activities.

To deal with the special problem of perceptions of conflict of interest that can arise in the course of clinical research activities, and particularly in the conduct of clinical trials, the committee made additional recommendations concerning the protocols by which university bodies review research proposals, especially proposals of clinical studies involving human subjects. First, the cover document, which must accompany any research grant proposal on its traverse through the university before it is released to a sponsoring agency, was modified by asking a new question: "Do any of the involved researchers have consulting arrangements, line management responsibilities, or substantial equity holdings in the proposed sponsor, vendor or subcontractor?"[11] If the answer to the question is "yes," then full explanation must be provided by the applicant.

Second, a new section entitled "Conflict of Interest" was added to the form entitled "Request for Institutional Approval of Project Involving Human Subjects at Risk," which states: "If materials being studied in the protocol will be supplied by commercial entities with which investigators consult or have financial interests, please identify this arrangement and respond to the following questions."[12] The questions are extensive and ask whether investigators or co-investigators have consulting agreements, equity interests, corporate employment relationships, and so on, with firms providing materials to be studied in the protocol. It is asked, "To what extent is the study driven by commercial interests as opposed to academic or patient care concerns?"; will graduate students, residents or other trainees be involved, and if so, how will their interests be protected?; is there any likelihood that the results of the study will not be made freely available? Furthermore, and particularly important, if consultative or financial relationships exist, those relationships must be disclosed fully on the consent form given to each potential subject for review and signature.

Although the ultimate onus for full disclosure continues to rest on the integrity of individual faculty/investigators, these changes in university policy and procedure have been important and beneficial. They have raised the sensitivities of all concerned, both applicants and members of institutional review bodies, to real and potential problems of conflict of interest, and they provide reasonable institutional safeguards that have proved to be compatible with the fragile ecology of the research university.

It is important to recognize--notwithstanding the Congressional rhetoric of the last few years--that for most of the past decade the federal government has been strongly promoting the transfer of technology and the commercialization of the fruits of the basic research that it supports. Thus, in 1980, the Stevenson-Wydler Technology Innovation Act and the Patents and Trademark Amendments of 1980 were enacted, both of which require universities to pursue vigorous programs of patenting and licensing for the commercial development of federally funded basic research. More recently, in 1986, Congress enacted the federal Technology Transfer Act, which provided similar exhortation to scientists working in federal laboratories. Biomedical scientists have indeed responded to these urgings; and, as one result, I believe the academic medical center presently faces problems of conflict of interest and commitment that are qualitatively different in important respects from those with which the research university has traditionally grappled. Some of these concerns may be exemplified by the following kinds of questions:

1. Will increasing commercial ties of academic biomedical scientists lead to restriction of scientific communication or of the sharing of research materials in a manner that will corrode collegial relationships and impair scientific progress?
2. Will such commercialization, and the fact of significant financial interest by faculty investigators, lead to inadvertent or advertent distortion in the conduct of science and the reporting of scientific results?
3. Will perceived or real conflicts undermine the role of the university as a credible, impartial, and disinterested societal resource? Does this commercialization of biomedical science threaten to impair or distort the educational experience of students and trainees, unduly influence the research directions and objects of faculty investigators, corrode their commitment to academic values, and challenge the fundamental expectation of faculty appointment--namely, that "faculty owe an overriding professional allegiance to the university"?[13]

Now, these several questions clearly are different in kind as well as in degree. With respect to those that concern blatant distortion of the conduct and reporting of research, it is my view that diligent attention to prevention (based on the promotion of high ethical standards) and to oversight (based on mechanisms of full and timely disclosure at all levels of the scientific enterprise) represents the most attractive and credible approach that does not violate the fundamental social contract between an academic institution and its faculty.

Much more perplexing, however, are the broader questions, which speak to the credibility of the university as a public trust for knowledge; to the disinterest of faculty investigators in selecting topics of scientific inquiry and pursuing them with impartiality, skepticism, and rigor; and to the corrosion of the principle of primary allegiance to the university, which is the principal, substantive contractual expectation that Stanford University makes of a member of its academic council. To this point, it is of interest to note that although Stanford's expectations of its faculty certainly embrace both teaching and scholarship, the university appears to lay particular and exclusive claim to a faculty member's teaching expertise and commitment--yet makes no comparably specific claim against the faculty member's scholarship. Thus, the single explicit proscription of outside faculty activity, beyond the broad and permissive language in the consulting policy, states that "Faculty members on regular duty, . . . regardless of their percentage of appointment, are normally not permitted to accept teaching appointments at other educational institutions."[14] That proscription speaks to what is a fundamental difference between the basic mission of a school of medicine and that of most of the other schools of the university.

Generally within the university, the allocation of resources and positions to academic units is principally determined by pedagogic objectives encompassed in teaching and scholarship. In most instances, there is a rough metric (expressed, for example, in the faculty-to-student ratio) that relates the numbers, distribution, and administrative organization of faculty slots not only to explicit scholarly objectives but to curricular obligations. Such a metric becomes extraordinarily attenuated in the staffing plan of the contemporary academic medical center. Recall that the very concept of "the academic medical center" as it has evolved in the US is relatively recent. It only reached full expression in the period immediately following World War II, which witnessed enormous growth in the numbers of faculty members working in university centers, who were appointed on a full-time basis, and were primarily recruited and rewarded on the basis of their potential and accomplishment in research. Admittedly, to be sure, medical school faculty are responsible for diverse teaching responsibilities, involving students and trainees at all levels of professional maturation; but if one examines the numbers and sizes of departments and the total numbers of full-time faculty in academic medical centers, one would be hard pressed to rationalize those numbers in any plausible way with student populations or units of teaching responsibility.

The full-time basis of faculty appointment is a defining characteristic of the academic medical center and is unique to the school of medicine among all the academic units on the Stanford University campus. Clearly, that basis was designed to mitigate, if not eliminate, the distraction of private clinical practice and clinical earnings and thereby to focus the energy--and the commitment--of this rapidly expanding cadre of faculty on the fundamental purposes of the university; that is, on the discovery, transmission, and conservation of knowledge. Thus, like the requirement of celibacy in the priesthood, the restriction of full-time faculty from private clinical practice was consciously imposed to foster a state of academic grace. But it is clear in retrospect that in attempting to secure such a primary academic commitment, the architects of the academic medical center were either not sufficiently prescient or not so much concerned with the potential distraction of outside activities relating to research.

Academic medicine is an undertaking that deals with conjoint products; and, accordingly, faculty are hired with the expectation that they will engage in multiple, conjoint activities that are difficult to separate into cleanly quantifiable, independent elements. Thus, we speak of conjoining the conduct of science with the training of scientists; patient care with clinical teaching and clinical investigation; the education of medical students and graduate students with future physicians and future biomedical investigators. But examined objectively, it seems clear that academic medical centers have developed so robustly in this nation primarily on the basis of research expectations and opportunities. Might one then suggest that in the employment of medical school faculty, it is not so much the commitment to deliver teaching for which one contracts "primary professional allegiance" as it is to deliver scholarship?

What is it about commercial-academic medical center entanglements that distinguishes them from the array of commercial relationships that may comfortably exist in other disciplines elsewhere in the university? The differences are of several kinds. First, it is a striking feature of contemporary biotechnology that the foundational knowledge base continues to reside largely within university laboratories. The work of the commercial laboratory, particularly in start-up companies, is often extraordinarily difficult to distinguish from that being conducted simultaneously in faculty laboratories. This feature is qualitatively different from the more typical circumstances of commercialization of faculty inventions, where the commercial work is truly developmental and is based on knowledge or technology that, from the perspective of the faculty inventor's continuing academic program, is "past history."

Second, the similarity and contemporaneity of commercial and academic research in biomedicine often leads to the further complication that the faculty inventor's participation is deemed mandatory to the viability of the commercial enterprise. Stanford University has for at least a decade adhered to a policy of "not going into business with its faculty" and has had a strong, if not absolute, aversion to the granting of exclusive licenses (especially prospective licenses) to start-up companies in which faculty inventors hold equity. However, the requirement by investors of active faculty participation in the launching of new commercial enterprises not only leads to discomfiture and confusion of faculty role and obligation, but it also tends fatally to undercut the licensing policy-- since a nonexclusive license without the close participation of the faculty inventor may often be veritably worthless.

A third distinctive feature of the commercialization of biomedical science, of course, is the common expectation that products to be forthcoming will prove useful (and valuable) in the diagnosis or treatment of human disease. In such circumstances, it is not only the involvement of the faculty inventor in launching the commercial enterprise that is of concern; the same faculty inventor often becomes an obligatory participant in the ensuing clinical evaluation of the putatively useful products that may be generated. This form of faculty entanglement in the conduct of clinical research and clinical trials is far more problematic than that arising from a faculty member's financial relationship to a company in which he/she is not a founder or an otherwise key scientific participant. For in the latter case, mandatory disclosure, or even voluntary disinvestment, can at least be contemplated to avoid the substance, or the appearance, of conflict; but, in the former instance, disclosure, even though mandatory, does not eliminate the problem of perceived (if not actual) conflict, and disinvestment is often expressly prohibited by the conditions of the commercial venture.

In our experience at Stanford, we have encountered a number of cases of this kind, brought voluntarily by faculty who were troubled by such confusion of roles and were searching for procedural remedies that would allow good and exciting science to proceed, while permitting them the preservation of their moral composure and ethical standards, as well as peace of mind. The working out of appropriate procedures is certainly possible, but it is not always simple or formulaic. To the contrary, it requires a high degree of customization to conform to the specifics of the particular case, and it must be flexible enough to respond to new and often complex kinds of conflict situations (perceived or actual) that cannot be managed by simple prohibitions or generic prescriptions.

In the past several years, many academic institutions, professional organizations, and the National Institutes of Health have given renewed attention to these issues of conflict. The Association of Academic Health Centers (AAHC) recently published a lengthy policy paper entitled "Conflicts of Interest in Academic Health Centers."[15] Almost concurrently, a shorter document was published by the Association of American Medical Colleges (AAMC) entitled "Guidelines for Dealing with Faculty Conflicts of Commitment and Conflicts of Interest in Research."[16] The two documents are different in focus, but entirely compatible with one another.

The AAHC report carefully defines conflicts of interest and commitment, puts them in a broad perspective, and emphasizes that such conflicts tend to be ubiquitous within the professions. Accordingly, and this is a very important point, it is naïve to think that conflict can be either totally prevented or eradicated. Instead, it must be recognized and managed, and in the view of the AAHC task force, the principal responsibility for those tasks rests squarely within academic institutions. The concluding section of the report posits some guiding principles and develops some general guidelines for resolving and managing conflicts of interest and commitment.

The first and overarching principle is that of primary commitment to the university. The document states that "a person who accepts a full-time appointment to the faculty, or full-time research position, where status is a full-time research fellow or student, has an obligation to devote his/her primary professional effort and allegiance to the university.... It is inappropriate for faculty or academic staff members, without prior approval, to divert to other entities or institutions opportunities for research, education, clinical care or financial support which otherwise might flow to the university." The report goes on to urge that "each university should develop policies that identify those activities which require prior approval and those for which disclosure is sufficient."

The next set of principles addresses disclosure: "Faculty, researchers, staff and students should be required upon initial affiliation, and periodically thereafter, to disclose significant financial, personal or professional relationships that raise a potential conflict of interest between their academic role and outside interests, as defined by university policies.... Significant financial, personal or professional relationships that raise a potential conflict of interest should be fully and accurately disclosed in all speeches, writings, advertising, public communications or collegial discussions relating to the sponsored research."

Another set of principles is concerned with the promotion of technology transfer and is based on the premise that the university has an obligation to ensure the dissemination of knowledge. The principles state that each university should have policies concerning patents and licensing. The next set of principles is concerned with the encouragement of the free exchange of information, "a fundamental value underlying the university's mission," and emphasizes the need to avoid restrictions on such information flow, whether those restrictions emanate from federal sponsors or from commercial sponsors interested in the protection of proprietary interests. Finally, there is a set of principles that deals with the necessary protections of students and research staff.

As noted, the report of the AAMC is entirely congruent with the AAHC document. Some illustrative excerpts from the AAMC publication are presented below:

> As the interface between research and commercial activities expands, faculty in our democratic society are confronted with often conflicting realities. On the one hand, the freedom to pursue one's own economic interests is guaranteed by our system of government and, indeed, is the driving force of our national economy. At the same time, the requirement for objectivity and commitment in biomedical and behavioral research dictates extreme care as scientists pursue research activities while also pursuing their own economic goals.... The opportunity for investigators to receive financial or other personal rewards from their endeavors is not intrinsically unacceptable, as long as it does not adversely influence the objectivity, integrity or professional commitment of an investigator.
>
> It is not possible to completely eradicate the potential for conflict of interest because there are certain rewards that are inherent in the structure of our research enterprise. Such rewards may be completely unrelated to

relationships with industry or private sponsorship. For example, positive research results per se may contribute to opportunities for publication, promotion, tenure, grant renewals, etc. In a sense, these influences can be as much a source of conflict in the search for truth as interests of a pecuniary nature. But kept in perspective, such incentives are not inherently bad and are indeed the motivating forces for diligent scientists.

There is no simple approach to dealing with conflicts of interest among faculty. The strategies for managing conflicts are just as numerous as the types of conflicts that may occur. It is important to be cognizant, however, that conflicts in research indeed will arise at some point in time. They are a natural product of the intersection of the vast matrix of faculty personal responsibilities and needs with the network of professional affiliations and activities that must be maintained. Conflicts are not necessarily unacceptable and many can be managed provided adequate mechanisms are in place for disclosure and oversight.[17]

For university officers, the key to successful resolution of the issues arising from these conflict situations is rooted in the three principles of personal integrity, primary allegiance, and full and timely disclosure. There must be diligence and sensitivity in managing instances of potential or real conflict on an individualized or customized basis within a broad framework of clear institutional policies; and effective approaches to these issues must inevitably be seasoned with generous dollops of common sense.

With respect to the admittedly amorphous but pivotal concept of primary allegiance, it is noteworthy that recently issued Harvard Medical Center guidelines on conflicts of interest and commitment approach problems of conflict by ordering activities into three different categories, those that are routinely allowable, those ordinarily allowable following disclosure, and those that "may be allowable only after disclosure, review and approval with oversight by a standing committee of the Harvard Medical Center."[18] Within this last category of activities--in addition to typical examples of problematic financial entanglements--there is the following additional example: "A faculty member conducting research, externally and to the disadvantage of the university or hospitals and their legitimate interests, that would ordinarily be conducted within the university or hospital."

That statement is of particular interest in its explicit extension of the university's concept of primary allegiance to faculty research, as well as to faculty teaching. The statement is fully in accord with the content of the first and overarching guiding principle in the AAHC document, and it provides a useful example that all research-intensive universities and academic medical centers might wish to consider with care.

Although the analysis, the philosophy, and the particular guidelines encompassed in the AAHC and AAMC reports may not serve to satisfy the most vociferous critics and overseers, the documents are thoughtful, helpful, and appropriate. It cannot be forgotten that the culture of the university is ultimately rooted in the assumption of personal integrity. There is no body of law or regulation that can provide absolute safeguards against failures or breaches of that integrity in the occasional individual instance; and any remedy that can be conjectured that purports to prevent or eradicate all vestiges of conflict will inevitably threaten an ominous assault on the essential fabric of academic life. In seeking solutions (and in attempting to manage these issues competently and effectively, especially in the glare of the public spotlight) it is essential that the delicate environment that has nurtured such remarkable scientific progress and enabled such gratifying returns on this nation's generous public investment in biomedical research not be irreparably damaged.

NOTES

1   D. Korn, "The Culture of the Research University," in *Project on Scientific Fraud and Misconduct* (report on workshop number 3) (Washington, DC: AAAS-ABA National Conference of Lawyers and Scientists, 1989).
2   *Conflicts of Interest in Academic Health Centers* (Washington, DC: Association of Academic Health Centers, 1990).
3   Association of American Medical Colleges (AAMC), "Guidelines for dealing with faculty conflicts of commitment and conflicts of interest in research," *Academic Medicine* 65, no.7 (1990):487-96.
4   *Conflicts of Interest*; AAMC, "Guidelines."
5   C.K. Gunsalus and J. Rowan, "You and the big U: protecting your interests and your name--conflict of interest considerations in spin-off licensing" (paper presented at the Second Conference on the University Spin-Off Corporation, Virginia Polytechnic Institute, Blacksburg, VA, May 1989).
6   Stanford University, *Research Policy Handbook* (Stanford, CA: Stanford University, 1989).
7   Korn, "The Culture of the Research University."
8   Stanford University, *Research Policy Handbook*.
9   *Ibid.*
10   *Ibid.*
11   *Ibid.*
12   *Ibid.*
13   *Ibid.*
14   Stanford University, *Faculty Handbook* (Stanford, CA: Stanford University, 1984).
15   *Conflicts of Interest*.
16   AAMC "Guidelines."
17   *Ibid.*
18   Harvard University Faculty of Medicine, *Policy on Conflicts of Interest and Commitment* (New Haven, CT: Harvard University, 1990).

14

Managing Conflict of Interest in Faculty, Federal Government, and Industrial Relations

Barbara C. Hansen and Kenneth D. Hansen

CONFLICTS OF INTEREST ARE UBIQUITOUS

With the growth of the biotechnology industry and vigorous application of the Technology Transfer Act, interactions between faculty and commercial firms have increased, particularly in the biomedical research area. Simultaneously, attention to issues of conflict of interest has grown, and public focus upon several well-publicized cases has increased concern about the potential effects of such conflicts.

Conflicts of interest in university-industry-government relationships come in a variety of forms and sizes. Consequently, appropriate measures for the management of one type of conflict might be inappropriate for another type of conflict. Some conflicts can be appropriately managed, others must be eliminated or prohibited, and still others are adequately handled by simple disclosure.

In the scientific research context, the most restrictive definition of conflict of interest refers to specific, substantial financial gain to be realized through research. For example, in the extreme situation, an individual might expect to gain substantial financial benefit with the finding of positive results and to suffer significant personal financial loss in the absence of such positive results. The existence of an implied fiduciary relationship--for example, between the investigator and the public (or other scientists)--is an essential component to the existence of conflict of interest. The question posed within that relationship is: are there extraneous interests that may have an untoward effect on the trust implied by the fiduciary relationship? The principal issue of concern to scientists should be the means by which the objectivity and reliability of research results can be assured.

THE NATURE OF CONFLICTS OF INTEREST IN UNIVERSITY-INDUSTRY-GOVERNMENT INTER-RELATIONSHIPS

Inherent Conflict of Interest

Academic scientists, like other professionals, have inherent conflicts of interests and conflicts of commitments. For example, there is an inherent bias toward success of any project undertaken. Bias exists to enhance opportunity for advancement in academic rank, increased salary, and academic reputation. Similar bias exists among those employed by government and industry. It is reasonable and prudent to simply assume the presence of such natural biases, and to rely upon further replication and validation to provide confidence in research findings.

Inherent conflicts arising from an employment relationship need not be circumscribed in any way. The time-honored practice of identifying the scientists involved in a publication by reference to their institution or employer and the sources of support for the research should serve to place the public on notice of potential biases. Disclosure, therefore, is the principal method for managing such inherent conflicts. In fact, such inherent conflicts generally need no specific mitigation, as they are readily apparent and their impact can be assessed by an observer (for example, when the president of a company speaks glowingly of the results of their own studies). Clearly, the most important individual in any conflict situation is the investigator. For it is only through the investigator's own actions that a conflict can lead to untoward outcomes.

Inherent conflict of interest due to the desire to reach a positive outcome in the conduct of a particular study must be assumed and is not necessarily detrimental. In fact, it can be the very motivation that leads a scientist to do one last experiment that ultimately proves to lead to a new discovery or a new application. It is the motivation that prevents the premature disposal of a potentially promising agent. It is the motivation to seek one more alternative dose or protocol, carry out one more test, and to therefore press the limits of science. Thus, the desire for a positive result may be the force that energizes science in the first place. Positive incentives produce direct financial gain through an increase in the value of equity, or may produce indirect financial gain through an enhanced reputation, honoraria, salary raises, or other rewards such as simple pride of discovery. In either case, science is best served by the energy that such motivations help to generate.

Induced Conflict of Interest

Induced conflicts of interest are by their nature changeable and temporary, and generally involve research support or other financial matters.

The award of research funds by either government or industry confers a bias to achieve favorable results such that the grantor will continue financial support or otherwise recognize the successful works of the grantee scientist. Honoraria, consulting contracts, and paid travel also may tend to bias the scientist in favor of a project.

We must be aware of, and sensitive to, the "swinging pendulum" nature of the university/industry relationship. Ever since the first company lured a scientist into a testing agreement, concerns have been raised about the potential for conflicts of various interests, and the potential effects of such industrial involvements (1) on the education process, for students or post-doctoral fellows involved in study; (2) on scientific communication due to confidentiality and proprietary interests; and (3) on the possible distortion of the topics studied by scientists under inducements of financial support offered through industry. It is not appropriate or useful to the public to seek to eliminate such concerns; but, rather, it is important to promote a continuing dialogue that enhances each scientist's awareness of and assessment of the potential effects of such motivations in their everyday behavior. In a scientific laboratory, where part of its support is industrial and part federal, each day constitutes a day of balancing priorities and motivations. There is nothing new in this balancing effort, nor anything inherently untoward about it. It is important that potential negative effects of such relationships are continually evaluated, and that scientists in such positions are well aware of such effects. In recent years, "conflicts of interest" have frequently been combined with discussions of "conflicts of commitment." This position recognizes that an academic investigator has many interests and many commitments, and balancing all of these is the challenge that must be met in order to assure the objectivity and trustworthiness of scientific output. To that scientist falls the responsibility of providing whatever controls or balancing protocols are needed to support the validity of any findings in the laboratory, be they supported by commercial interests or by public funds.

Induced conflicts can be handled according to the magnitude of the potential bias that can be inferred. It may be necessary to set some threshold, below which no disclosure is necessary. Even those most inclined to regulate science would agree that *de minimis* honoraria, for example, would normally have little impact on the honesty of science.

Absolute Conflict of Interest

While it is beyond the purview of this chapter, there can be situations wherein the conflict of interest is so great as to preclude careful and reliable scientific inquiry. Any bribe, illegal contract, duress, or extortion is such an example.

SCIENTIFIC QUALITY ASSURANCE

Conflict-of-interest issues should not be confused with scientific quality assurance. The scientific method coupled with ongoing peer review has served us well in maintaining the quality of science. While examples exist of conflict-induced unethical behavior resulting in falsification of data, such cases have usually become apparent during further scientific inquiry and peer review. No external rule of conduct will ensure personal honesty.

MANAGEMENT OF CONFLICT OF INTEREST

The Appearance of Conflict

It is unfortunate that some writers have suggested that even the appearance of conflict of interest must be avoided. We find such a stance to be inappropriate and clearly not in the best interest of science or the public good. "Appearance of conflict" is in the eye of the beholder. Virtually any human endeavor could be painted to be unethical or at least self-serving. For example, the subject chosen by a sculptor may not have been chosen primarily for its artistic value, but may have been chosen for its potential for remuneration. Does that in itself make the quality of the art less valuable, or less important?

Scientists must constantly make decisions that affect the potential continued funding of their research, whether federally or privately supported. The fact that some investigators may choose to undertake a commercially viable research project while also being supported by funds from the federal government can be viewed by some as a conflict-of-interest problem, and by others as a strength. It is neither possible nor appropriate to attempt to resolve such differences of opinion, but rather it is important to recognize and to accept that all such views should be considered. Investigators must be free to balance many diverse motivations in the selection of topics, and in the methods of research. In fact, such diversity of opinion and of action needs strengthening, not lessening.

At risk is the possibility of compromising scientific objectivity and of bias in professional judgment. That possibility exists in virtually all aspects of science and of life. We will limit this chapter to management of conflict of interest as it appears in academic-research situations. The current climate of dialogue concerning issues of conflict of interest is, for the most part, positive. There is no doubt that this dialogue promotes attention to ethical standards and enhanced sensitivity to the public view of research activities.

As noted before, appropriate and necessary disclosure is the cornerstone of conflict-of-interest management. But, what exactly is to be disclosed; and, once it is disclosed, what is the individual or group to do with the information? Perhaps, as with academic misconduct, gradations of conflicts of interest should now be considered.

Let us examine an example of possible conflict of interest, and then modify the example to develop variants in nature and degree of apparent conflict. For example, an academic scientist is flown to the headquarters of a pharmaceutical company to give a scientific lecture and is provided with an honorarium (say,

$2,000 dollars) for both the presentation of the research seminar and a day of consultation with scientists of the company, in the scientist's area of expertise. Should the investigator report the honorarium or the relationship with the pharmaceutical firm when the results of the federally funded university-based research are reported? Most scientists would say "no." Nevertheless, one of the elements of conflict of interest exist: The scientist has benefited personally and financially from the research. When the research was carried out, the investigator knew (or should have known) that positive results would be of substantial interest to pharmaceutical firms. Consider the further case in which the industrial consultation took place after the first oral presentation of the results at a scientific meeting (considered "confidential scientific discussions between scientists"), but prior to submission of a full manuscript to a refereed journal. Has one company gained an advantage through the early "purchase" of new information by this honorarium? Even something so simple as providing a scientific seminar to a pharmaceutical firm can be fraught with appearance of conflicts and possible untoward motivations. Despite such concerns, regulatory approaches have little role in mediating such interactions.

Perhaps the most legitimate bounds to the disclosure process should be a threshold of "substantial involvement" or "significant financial risk or benefit." In most potential conflict-of-interest situations, even disclosure itself would be unnecessary since the amounts of time and/or financial remuneration involved fall into the category of "trivial."

In some situations, it may be appropriate and perhaps even necessary for scientists to enter into a profit-sharing arrangement over a device or discovery made or developed in an academic or publicly supported laboratory. This may be essential to the further development of the discovery to the point of potential commercialization. The scientist (for example, Thomas Edison) finds it necessary to invest personal resources in return for long-range potential profits through equity holdings and may even involve investments by friends and relatives in return for equity. Such equity involvement, in fact, more often results in losses than in profits.

Other profit-sharing arrangements may result from formal licensing agreements, wherein a license fee is paid or a royalty is arranged on the potential sales of the product. Further consultation for a fee may be required on an ongoing basis. In fact, such consultation may be critical to the further commercial development of a product. The fledgling venture may even provide research support to the original developer, and such investment may be both a good business judgment and scientifically important.

Profits can also be realized by an academic scientist through the direct sale of a product, either manufactured "in his garage" or with his employer's facilities and encouragement. It is interesting that one journal editor has strongly espoused the view that scientists should not hold equity interest in any area of science with which they deal. This is tantamount to saying to a businessman, "you may drill for oil, but you cannot own wells," or "you may not buy and sell stock in any field of human endeavor in which you have personal expertise." It seems unconscionable that well-meaning individuals have generalized these actions into a broad area of prohibition, under the assumption that such buying and selling (de facto) would be unethical or immoral. There are very specific laws concerning "insider trading." As one biotechnology firm recently discovered, those laws can be strongly enforced through legal action. Illegal behavior on the part of scientists or anyone else is just that: illegal! It is certainly likely that scientists, working with pharmaceutical firms, will develop a general idea of which firms are best managed, most sound scientifically; and, therefore, at least by some estimates, most likely to produce a profit to shareholders. Scientists should not be prohibited from such analyses of the stock market on the basis of the profession they choose to follow. There is clearly a major difference between insider trading and well-informed investment judgments. One is prohibited; the other is not, and should not be.

This does not mean, however, that there are not some highly circumscribed situations in which an equity holding might be a matter of significant and reasonable public concern and, in fact, may need to be prohibited. For example, during, and for a reasonable period (perhaps one year) following, participation in a phase III clinical trial, it might be appropriate to prohibit buying and selling activities on the part of involved investigators in the related firms. Such an approach would not require an investigator to sell all pharmaceutical equity holdings held prior to the initiation of such a trial, and therefore, would not prohibit the possibility of profiting from the outcome of the research--that is, from positive findings. This might be permissible, however, only if the broader scientific process has been well-protected via the involvement, for example, of other investigators without such equity holdings. Equity holdings per se do not necessarily create a problem, but must be considered in the context of the overall clinical trial, and with consideration given to the overall economic advantages potentially accruable to an investigator on the basis of the trial.

Spin offs from federally or commercially supported research may potentially have commercial value and lead to personal profit. For example, a computer program developed during the course of a federal grant project might be contracted out to a commercial firm. Or lacking such interest, the program might be invested in by the originator for further development of the "user-friendly interface," and documentation. This further testing and refinement might ultimately result in a significant commercial success. Clearly, it is in the interest of the initial program developer to see the program developed for wide commercial use. In fact, the investigator may also prove to be the best salesman for the product, either overtly or more subtly through the publication of his research using the computer program. Should such work be prohibited? This would not be in the best interest of science or of the public. Indeed, if the program were not to be commercially developed, many investigators would find it impossible to use this tool without further substantial repetitious and costly investment. Thus, the product of one person's intellect would be limited in its use with little benefit to the public. Recognizing the importance of such technology transfer for the public good, in fact, the federal government has passed several pieces of legislation encouraging this process.

Finally, increased financial remuneration can come indirectly through career advancement and influence in the scientific community. A scientist's "independent judgments" and objectivity can be influenced by many different forms of financial and nonfinancial reward. These are not issues of contention nor issues to be managed, but exist instead to heighten sensitivity and awareness.

Conflict-of-interest management processes should be designed so as not to find things to prohibit, but rather so as to develop innovative ways for mitigating such potentially negative effects toward the long-range goal of supporting public needs for biomedical science and the improvement of health. Thus, despite the growth in the 1980s of academic-industry collaborative efforts, studies, on balance, point to more positive than negative effects of this effort.[1] Risk-benefit analyses are warranted and should assist in keeping the dialogue active concerning appropriate balances in these relationships.

We must have significant concern about well-meaning efforts aimed at "eliminating" or wiping out conflicts of interest. The potential problems identified in the public outcry following the issuance of the NIH/ADAMHA Proposed Guidelines for Policies on Conflict of Interest (1989) were exceptionally strong.[2] Industry and academia were united, as were many of the scientific and academic associations, in opposing the proposed guidelines, which were thought to be far in excess of those needed to mediate potential conflicts of interest. An analysis of risks versus benefits showed that the preponderance of views indicated concern that success of such efforts to eliminate conflict of interest through application of those guidelines would have resulted in the substantial loss of benefits to the public. Perhaps most troubling was the guidelines' apparent lack of trust in the judgment and behavior of scientists. That lack of trust unfortunately was fueled by an occasional case of significant abuse, and by the Congressional and media interest in such cases. Nevertheless, the research arms of the federal government must be cautious in accepting pressures such as these, for while seemingly innocent and well intended, such actions clearly are not "risk free."

Mitigation of the Effects of Conflicts of Interest
The greatest concern for conflict-of-interest situations should be directed to those situations where the study itself and its results cannot be readily replicated, or are not being concurrently studied by other independent laboratories. Under such situations, the ability to question the results can be compromised; and, thus, the discovery of any deleterious effects of conflict might be more difficult.

There are, however, many situations in which any potential untoward effects of existing conflicts of interest can be identified and/or mitigated. When a conflict-of-interest situation arises, it is appropriate to analyze systematically the means--despite the conflict--by which objectivity in the scientific process can be ensured. Scientifically valid and important means already exist in the repertoire of scientists' activities. Such situations or counter-balancing conditions of study design or implementation to assure or promote objectivity in the face of conflicts of interest might include:

1. The existence of simultaneous studies by other investigators who do not share the same conflict of interest;
2. Blinding of a protocol to those directly involved in the collection of the data (for example, where the identity of the test agents are coded);
3. Analysis or secondary analysis of results by a "nonconflicted" party;
4. Audits of findings and results;
5. Limitation or insulation from the direct financial outcomes, such as by use of a blind trust;
6. Establishing outcome variables that are objective (the more objective and measurable, the less subject to untoward effects of conflict);
7. The availability of data for secondary analysis and interpretation;
8. "Double blind" controlled trials with random treatments;
9. Limiting discretion by the investigator (that is, concerning decisions on the inclusion or exclusion of subjects).

It has been suggested that conflicts of interest should be eliminated except when the conflict itself represents an "overriding social benefit." Such a standard cannot and should not be promulgated. It unbalances the situation of risk/ benefit analysis to one of potentially low risk, low benefit. Such a regulatory approach would inappropriately limit individual or scientific freedom in the interest of some undefined social benefit assignable to the "absence of risk," a condition which could, in fact, be counter to the public interest.

The situation of a major clinical trial should be viewed as a special condition, and generalizations from that model are inappropriate. The example of the well-publicized clinical study in which participants in the study committed themselves to neither buy nor sell, nor hold stock nor equity, in the companies involved, nor to accept consultation fees from the same companies during the course of the study, was appropriate and might be more generally applicable to such large-scale clinical trials. However, it would not be appropriate to the vast majority of research circumstances for which neither risk nor benefit would warrant such prohibitions.[3] When a number of people are assembled in order to have the advantage of their joint wisdom, inevitably assembled with those people, are all of their prejudices, their passions, their errors of opinion, their local interests and their selfish views. Or, as aptly phrased by Ben Franklin, "From such an assembly, can a perfect product be expected?"[4] It is clear that the basic scientist or clinical investigator must remain the principal party responsible for the assessment and management of conflicts of interest. When a group is involved in collaborative research, it is important that the group share an understanding of any conflicts and biases in various members of the group. This is as much a part of collaborative study as is understanding of any other biases that an investigator brings to the table.

One of the issues that must be considered in relying heavily on "peer review" of disclosures is the fact that those who are uninvolved in industrial relationships have little understanding of their complexity and their importance. Indeed, those with no commercial involvement are far more likely to find themselves in the position of "prohibiting" all or most such financial interactions. Likewise, a peer group made up only of those with substantial commercial involvement raises concern that scrutiny may be inadequate. For any sort of conflict-of-interest review process to gain credibility with the investigators and, therefore, to be used and supported, an appropriately balanced process of judgment that clearly recognizes and is generally supportive of commercial involvement by faculty is critical. Without a credible process, creative forces will produce other alternative methods to reach the same end, and proscriptions concerning disclosure would become mute.

As one protection against untoward interpretation and proscriptions concerning conflicts of interest, an investigator would be wise to provide for himself (or herself) and his collaborators, documentation of such decisions involving relationships with commercial companies. Such documentation or recognition of potential conflicts is in itself evidence of cognizance of the potential for a problem or the appearance thereof.

Should universities or government agencies enter into this scenario? Should micromanagement, the production of "dos" and "do nots," or the specification of guidelines become the norm?

University practices, in relation to conflict of interest, have been evolving slowly over the past ten years. Most universities request or require disclosure of potential financial conflicts of interest. Some have implemented various review processes. Nevertheless, the institutional processes are in their infancy in this area. There are clearly examples of failure of some universities to provide adequate protections, and the policies of other institutions have not been tested, and will probably not withstand the test of time when multiple situations are examined. There are clearly certain situations that require scrutiny and perhaps ongoing monitoring, but may not require prohibition. For example, part-time service as a manager in a small company, or the board of directors of a large company, could be compatible with university service as a faculty member. Special scrutiny of such roles and relationships might, however, be appropriate.

Promulgation of standards would clearly be premature at this time, and perhaps may prove unnecessary and unwarranted.

WHAT DOES THE FUTURE HOLD?

One of the positive outcomes of the present dialogue process concerning conflicts of interest will be the development and public availability of more and more examples of methods by which such potential conflicts have been mitigated and managed. We need a larger repertoire of means by which scientists, while enhancing university/industry relations, can simultaneously provide greater assurance to the public of the integrity of their work. Human judgments must come into play and those judgments will be made by many parties--colleagues, competitors, reporters, Congressional aides, and, yes, the involved scientist. It is unlikely that such judgments by such a diverse group will always be in accord. Where discord exists, it will be helpful over the coming years to analyze the nature of the discordant judgments and to work further toward understanding the motivations and biases of each party. With the further analysis of risk-benefit ratios, what seems to be evolving is a clearer and clearer picture of situational ethics. Conflicts of interest by some individuals may warrant outright prohibition. For example, the holding of equity by an FDA regulator involved in the assessment and approval of a product clearly has greater public importance than equity-holding by a scientist in a company supporting his research, where that stock had been purchased by his deceased grandfather! It is clear that as this process develops, thresholds of unacceptable conflict will become more apparent. For example, an equity-holding or financial arrangement involving less than $10,000 (or less than $100,000) might be of minimal concern and require mere disclosure to a supervisor. Further, the holding of a patent with a license arrangement might be minimally problematic even where the licensee is also supporting further developmental work on the product in the laboratory of the inventor.

Clearly, it is important for scientists, no matter what the issue, to continually scrutinize their own honesty and the degree to which their various commitments and motivations enter into the objective development of the soundest scientific outcomes. Such situations provide dilemmas that are a fact of life for many investigators. Attending to them, being alert to them, and dialoguing over them is important. We would, however, urge care in elevating such ethical dilemmas to a point where scientists could be significantly inhibited in their actions and interactions. It is our view that constant vigilance is the price of scientific freedom, but that prescriptions and proscriptions, except in highly delimited, high-risk situations must be assiduously avoided.

NOTES

1   D. Blumenthal, M. Gluck, K. Louis, *et al.*, "University-Industry Research Relationships in Biotechnology: Implications for the University," *Science* 232 (1986):1361-66; D. Blumenthal, M. Gluck, K. Louis, *et al.*, "Industrial Support of University Research in Biotechnology," *Science* 231 (1986):242-31; C.K. Gunsalus and J. Brown, "Conflict of Interest in the University Setting: I Know it When I See It," *Research Management Review* (Fall 1989):13-25.
2   For policies on conflict of interest, see: NIH *NIH Guide* 18, no.32 (15 September 1989).
3   B. Healy, L. Campeau, R. Gray, *et al.*, "Conflict of Interest Guidelines for a Multicenter Clinical Trial of Treatment after Coronary-Artery Bypass-Graft Surgery," *New England Journal of Medicine* 320 (1989):9551.
4   Benjamin Franklin at the Constitutional Convention on 15 September 1887.

15

Conflict-of-Interest Issues Surrounding Faculty Participation in, and Ownership of, Technology and Drug Companies

William B. Neaves and Kern Wildenthal

This chapter reflects issues considered over the last seven years at the University of Texas Southwestern Medical Center during the development and implementation of a new technology transfer program, partially funded by the John A. Hartford Foundation. The centerpiece of the program is a private, for-profit corporation called Dallas Biomedical Corporation.[1] Created with $12 million of investment capital, its primary purpose is to make money for stockholders by transferring technology from research at Southwestern Medical Center to companies capable of manufacturing and marketing medical products. The medical center views the program as a way to help faculty scientists realize the practical public benefits of their research, without abandoning their university position or foregoing their fair share of financial returns.

Dallas Biomedical was structured to provide a source of funds to carry mature projects beyond basic research toward product development, and to offer a wider range of commercialization options, including the formation of new start-up companies. Dallas Biomedical assumes all business management rights in sponsored projects and splits all returns, including equity in new start-up companies, fifty-fifty with Southwestern Medical Center. Southwestern in turn splits its share of all returns fifty-fifty with the faculty member responsible for the project. No employee of Southwestern Medical Center can be a stockholder, officer, director, or employee of Dallas Biomedical Corporation, but both Southwestern and members of its faculty can receive equity in new companies founded by Dallas Biomedical, in return for transferring technology to them through agreements approved by the university administration and governing board.

CONFLICT OF INTEREST

Two aspects of conflicting interest can be distinguished.[2] One relates to how the faculty member spends time and effort. The other concerns how the faculty member's mind is oriented; that is, does another interest conflict with the conduct of unbiased research? The first kind of conflicting interest, sometimes described as conflicting commitment, is subject to relatively simple remedies. Keeping a professor on campus four days a week is easy if the university has the will to enforce traditional consulting guidelines. Keeping the professor's attention focused on university business is more difficult, especially if the professor has a significant stake in an outside venture. Until 1985, the University of Texas governed this kind of conflict of interest by denying faculty the right to own shares of stock in companies that might benefit from their research. This policy protected both the university and the public from professorial venality, but it also penalized both by inhibiting entrepreneurial inventiveness and by diminishing the motivation of faculty scientists to develop and improve products that might otherwise be successfully commercialized. Six years ago, the University of Texas changed its policy on equity ownership to accommodate the new technology transfer plan, developed by Southwestern Medical Center with Hartford Foundation support. The critical element in the new policy was equal sharing between the university and the faculty member in the financial rewards of commercialization. This included equal sharing of equity in new start-up companies based on technology arising from the faculty member's research.

REWARDING DEVELOPERS OF TECHNOLOGY WITH EQUITY

Emergence of the biotechnology industry over the last two decades coincided with the flowering of venture capitalism in the US. Smart money sought early-stage investment opportunities that offered a chance for substantial returns sooner than could be anticipated through the purchase of shares in established businesses. In contrast to the large, publicly held drug companies that preferred to rely on their own scientific staff to develop new products, venture capitalists worked readily with university faculty to found new companies based on product ideas arising from faculty members' research.

University faculty found it much easier to excite venture capital investors in new companies with their ideas than to generate enthusiasm among corporate giants. Unlike established drug companies that would occasionally negotiate with university faculty to license a desirable technology in exchange for a royalty interest in future sales, venture capitalists offered faculty scientists shares in the ownership of new companies. Venture capitalists preferred granting equity rather than royalty to owners of promising new technology for two reasons. First, venture investors often expected to realize the largest financial return in the shortest time through early sale of the new company to an established corporation seeking either to eliminate competition in the same field or to diversify into a new area, and marketing of the new company was facilitated if its products were unencumbered by royalty interests. Second, venture capitalists believed that equity ownership would prove more motivational than royalty in acquiring technology from faculty scientists and in securing their help in successfully transferring technology to new companies. The fact that a few faculty scientists have been enriched over the last decade by equity holdings in new biotechnology companies has reinforced the perceived advantage of equity over royalty.

ALIGNMENT OF INTERESTS

Although universities and businesses may enter mutually beneficial relationships, including cooperation in the formation and ownership of new companies, their fundamental interests and motives are different. Universities serve society by pursuing objective knowledge in an open forum and sharing it widely. Businesses seek to enrich shareholders by making profits and withholding proprietary information if necessary. Both generate public benefits, but they do so through the pursuit of very different goals. Individual faculty members can be pulled between these divergent interests, and if the conflict is unresolved, business and university may lose. The following example illustrates an unfortunate outcome for both institutions.

A molecular biologist on a medical school faculty developed a practical method of introducing and expressing foreign genes in mammalian cells. Although the potential medical applications of the technology were obvious, established corporations showed little interest in licensing the work. The scientist turned to venture capital firms with experience in biotechnology start-ups, and an agreement was soon reached to found a company based on the new method. In exchange for rights to the technology, the company offered the medical school and the scientist substantial shares of equity. Although the medical school eventually negotiated a technology license with the company, an institutional policy prevented both the school and its faculty from holding equity in a company doing business related to university research. The scientist resigned from the faculty, received equity, and accepted a senior position in the company. The medical school lost a talented and creative researcher, who soon devoted all available time and energy to the management of a fledgling business. The company lost valuable time bringing a product to market by relying on a senior member of the management team who lacked training and experience in running a business. Both organizations would have been better off if the scientist had remained in the medical school, teaching and conducting research, and a business professional had been recruited to manage the company.

Academic scientists whose research yields new product opportunities should not have to leave the university in order to hold equity in a company engaged in developing these products. Nor should a university be restricted to holding only a royalty interest in products arising from research conducted by its faculty. If the prospect of a fair return favors equity over royalty in a given situation, both the individual and the institution should be able to own stock shares issued in exchange for transferring technology to a company. Under most circumstances, the inventor and the university should share equally in stock shares allocated under the terms of a license agreement between the university and the company. By receiving equity together, the university and the faculty member enter a business relationship with their interests aligned rather than in potential conflict. The university sanctions the relationship by its participation and discourages any misapprehension that faculty involvement in commercialization of research results is suspect or inappropriate. By accepting an equity position, the university also places itself in a position to manage the relationship with the company, both for itself and on behalf of the faculty member. Because of accountability to other members of its faculty, to its governing board, and to society, the university serves as a credible guardian of public interest as it participates in the business relationship alongside the involved faculty member. So long as the equity position assumed by the university is fully revealed, the intense scrutiny brought to bear on the university by other members of its faculty will ensure that resources, such as space and personnel, are not misused to benefit the company. Similarly, by knowing who on its faculty holds equity in the company, the university can be alert to any inappropriate expenditure of faculty effort on behalf of the company. Essential to the university's role as a credible guardian of public interest, however, is the strict requirement that its administrative officers be precluded from personally owning shares or receiving any other remuneration from the company in which the university holds equity. The credibility of the university would be destroyed if the individuals administering its affairs were themselves perceived as having a personal financial stake in the company. Equally essential is the requirement for full disclosure, both by individual faculty members and by the university. For a faculty member, this means letting university administration and immediate supervisors know about equity held in companies related to the faculty member's research. For the university, it means public acknowledgement of ownership of company stock received in exchange for technology.

REMUNERATIVE ALTERNATIVES TO EQUITY

Before the convergence of biotechnology and venture capitalism brought equity to prominence, university scientists relied principally on royalty payments to reward inventiveness. In contrast to equity, which allows the scientist to benefit financially from the potential of an invention, royalty only pays for proven performance in the market over an extended period of time. This important distinction provides the basis for resolving some conflict situations. In a case where ownership of a company's shares could create the appearance of conflict, substitution of royalty for equity may satisfy the concern. The following example demonstrates this. Two medical school scientists developed a promising new therapy for leukemia. In the absence of support from an established drug company, they personally assumed the considerable burden of securing FDA approval for phase I clinical trials and funded these trials with research grants. The phase I trials showed that their new therapy had no toxic side effects, and several terminal patients experienced remission under the influence of the experimental drug. They made plans for phase II clinical trials, but the scale of this next step required a new and larger source of funds, so they turned to a venture capitalist in the local business community. Although venture capital had funded a number of successful high-technology companies in their community, none involved biotechnology or drug therapy. As a result, the community lacked experienced professionals who knew how to secure FDA approvals and conduct clinical trials, and who might be recruited to staff a new drug company. National venture capital groups declined the opportunity to pioneer a new industry in their community. Local investors eventually capitalized the new company and undertook the recruitment of professional staff from elsewhere in the country. In the meantime, the founding scientists could not abandon the phase II clinical trials until the new company hired knowledgeable staff to assume this responsibility. Their medical school, which owned the patents and know-how they had developed, received a substantial block of shares in the new company, but the continued participation of the founding scientists in clinical trials precluded their acceptance of equity in the new company, in exchange for transferring the technology underlying the new therapy. Instead, the scientists received a royalty interest in the sale of products the company would develop on the basis of their patents.

Should scientists be excluded from any involvement in the clinical testing of their inventions? Their participation may be desirable and permissible if their involvement is fully disclosed and adequate provision is made for independent recruitment of patients and evaluation of test results. Otherwise, the absence of suitable staff in a new company could delay or prevent the development of innovative drugs and deny the public effective new therapies. Can scientists who remain involved in clinical trials retain a remunerative interest in resulting products? This may depend on whether equity or royalty is involved.

For scientists participating in clinical testing of their invention, why should royalty be an ethically acceptable alternative to equity? By receiving a percentage of net sales over a product's commercial lifetime, an inventor bets on the product's long-term survival in an efficient marketplace. An inventor holding royalty interest has little financial incentive to skew results while the product's effectiveness undergoes premarket testing. A product that does not ultimately perform as advertised is unlikely to enrich an inventor through royalty payments.

Equity, on the other hand, might be liquidated at a substantial mark-up far in advance of actual product sales. The perceived value of ownership shares in a new company could be driven up sharply by biased results of premarket tests of its product. Hence, a financial incentive to skew test results could motivate an equity holder, whereas an inventor holding a royalty interest should find little to gain from introducing bias into product trials.

OTHER CONSIDERATIONS THAT MOTIVATE SCIENTISTS

Conflict-of-interest guidelines emphasize safeguards against financial inducements that might bias research. The general public understands venality in terms of tangible benefits ordinarily measured in dollars. Although continued public confidence in science and medicine demands that institutions adopt policies designed to prevent monetary interests from skewing the results of research, everyone should recognize that factors other than money may divert a scientist, if only unconsciously, from the objective pursuit of truth. Compared to the approbation of academic peers, promotion to tenure, election to prestigious societies, nomination for competitive awards, and infatuation with a particular theory, financial reward may be the least of a number of considerations that can potentially color an individual scientist's work. This may be especially likely in the case of clinical scientists who have shown some disregard for remuneration by electing to work full-time as members of a medical school faculty. Any number of nonpecuniary motives constitute a human variable in research that can only be eliminated through the replication of results in the hands of other investigators. If a piece of research is important enough to be the basis of a new product, other scientists will attempt to reproduce it, and they will tend to bring an attitude of healthy skepticism to the endeavor. The public's confidence in research is ultimately justified by the self-correcting nature of science.

BIAS IN RESEARCH

Important differences distinguish bias from fraud. Fraud may be said to occur when available facts support a judgement of intentional deceit. Highly publicized scandals notwithstanding, most scientists reasonably believe that fraudulent research is relatively uncommon. Bias, on the other hand, affects most scientists, since human beings inevitably harbor attitudes and prejudices that influence how they think about what they observe. Bias does not imply an intent to deceive. Indeed, researchers may even be quite unaware of a bias that colors their work. To safeguard against bias in research, both the scientist performing the work and the scientist's supervisors must be alert to potential sources of bias. Any number of nonpecuniary motives that may bias research can be assumed to influence all academic scientists to a greater or lesser degree, but monetary motives are not automatically expected to be part of the potential considerations shaping the work of a typical academic scientist. This is why full disclosure of financial interests is so necessary.

CONCLUSION

By aligning its interests with those of a faculty member in sharing ownership of a new business based on the faculty member's research, the university assumes a heightened obligation to protect the public. A policy requiring full disclosure of the university's equity holding is necessary, but not sufficient. It should be combined with scrutiny of the ongoing relationship between the university and related businesses by a standing committee of disinterested faculty and public representatives. Institutional review boards that oversee research involving human subjects provide a model for the composition and conduct of such a committee. A consensus of informed peers and lay people can best determine if the facts of a situation threaten the public's interest in unbiased research.

NOTES

1   R.L. Gatz, D.A. Scantland, and C.D. Minshall, "The Dallas Approach to Commercializing University Research," *Bio/Technology* 3 (1985):695-99.
2   M.J. Jackson, D.A. Blake, W.T. Butler, *et al.*, "Guidelines for Dealing with Faculty Conflicts of Commitment and Conflicts of Interest in Research," *Academic Medicine* 65 (1990):489-96; D. Korn, K. Wildenthal, G.N. Burrow, *et al.*, *Conflicts of Interest in Academic Health Centers* (Washington DC: Association of Academic Health Centers, 1990), 1-62.

16

Cooperation Between Academia and Industry: Opportunities and Challenges

Barbara Mishkin

Just as with other issues that have affected the research community (for example, research with human subjects, animal research, and scientific fraud), "conflicts of interest" as an issue of public policy has followed a predictable course in Washington. First, there were a few highly publicized "abuses" that led to congressional hearings--which further publicized and expanded on the original incidents. Next, the National Institutes of Health (NIH) issued proposed guidelines or draft regulations to assure Congress (and the rest of the country) that it had everything under control and that legislative action would not be necessary. Then, the scientific/academic communities responded with alarm, warning that the proposed rules--if adopted--would seriously impair their ability to pursue research, and that the negative consequences for the public's health would be significant. Finally, a resolution was achieved through the collaborative efforts of NIH and representatives of the communities to be regulated.

We have entered the phase of trying to achieve a consensus on conflicts of interest, but it will not be easy because of the tension between two public policies. One policy encourages cooperation between academe and industry, while the other warns that the objectivity of biomedical researchers can be contaminated by personal or financial interests. Yet cooperative ventures have been accepted in other parts of the academic community for decades, particularly in agriculture, engineering, and chemistry.[1]

Cooperative activities go back at least to 1862, when Congress granted large tracts of land to each state, to be sold to establish perpetual endowment funds for colleges "to teach such branches of learning as are related to agriculture and the mechanic arts . . . in order to promote the liberal and practical education of the industrial classes in the several pursuits and professions in life."[2] Consistent with this practical purpose, Congress required annual reports prepared by these "land grant colleges" to describe "any improvements and experiments made, with their cost and results, and such other matters, including State industrial and economical statistics, as may be supposed useful."[3]

Even in the elite, private schools of New England, relationships between university faculty and industry were established without apparent concern about conflicts of interest. For example, at the turn of the century, Alexander Graham Bell began a lengthy collaboration with Charles Cross, who served as a consultant to the Bell Telephone Company while also chairing the physics department at MIT.[4] This was not unusual in the fields of chemistry and engineering. Indeed, by 1968, 168 new companies had been founded by MIT faculty alone.[5]

During World War II, penicillin and corticosteroids were developed and commercialized through cooperative efforts involving the US government, the pharmaceutical industry, and academia.[6] More recently, collaboration between Merck, Sharp & Dohme, several agencies within the Public Health Service, and researchers based in academia resulted in the development, testing, and manufacturing of a safe and effective hepatitis vaccine.[7]

In biotechnology, cooperative arrangements between academia and industry have generated 400 new companies, and over 200 supply firms, while over 200 established firms have expanded into new fields.[8] Benefits of these collaborations accrue not only to local economies, but also to the health of our citizens. For example, American physicians now have access to over 400 diagnostic tools that are based upon biotechnology, and they have purer drugs and biologicals (such as human insulin and growth hormone) to administer to their patients.[9]

The participating institutions as well as the public at large benefit from such collaborations. Speaking at Congressional hearings in 1982, Donald Senich (Director of the National Science Foundation's Division of Industrial Science and Technological Innovation) described the major benefits as follows:

> First, these programs leverage federal funds, . . . second, [they] provide continuity of funding, strengthening academic departments, and enhancing graduate student and postdoctoral training. Third, cooperation ensures job opportunities for graduates of the participating universities, at the same time enhancing the transfer of knowledge embodied in these graduates to industry. Last, but not least, cooperation does enhance information exchange between universities and industry.[10]

The opportunities for industry include direct and continuing access to some of most creative research talent in the country; use of research facilities, equipment, and personnel (including principal investigators, students, postdoctoral students, and technicians); and notice of (as well as the right to develop) breakthroughs in science and technology.

Recently, however, collaboration between academia and industry has been challenged, particularly as to the propriety of having products tested by the researchers who developed them or who have a financial stake in their commercial success. A primary concern is the potential for bias (real or perceived) that is introduced when scientists who conduct research to determine the safety and efficacy of new products have financial interests that depend on the outcome of their evaluations.[11]

There is also concern that the need of industrial sponsors to protect proprietary interests may conflict with the traditional goals of academic institutions: to seek and freely disseminate new knowledge, to maintain objectivity and integrity in research, and to permit faculty and students to establish and pursue their own research goals without interference.[12] Some commentators fear that commercial sponsors will seek to delay publication of scientific articles--or even of PhD theses--in order to protect patentable interests; others suggest that faculty who are supported by industrial sponsors may pressure students to concentrate their research efforts in commercially promising areas, rather than permitting them to pursue their own research interests.[13] The White House, Congress, and administrative agencies have taken different and sometimes conflicting stands on the issues, resulting in uncertainty as to what the government really wants.

ENCOURAGING JOINT VENTURES AND
OTHER FORMS OF COOPERATION

Recent Federal Legislation

Congress passed the Stevenson-Wydler Technology Innovation Act in 1980 to enhance technology transfer and to maintain priority in international competition.[14]

Many new discoveries and advances in science occur in universities and Federal laboratories, while the application of this new knowledge to commercial and useful public purposes depends largely upon actions by business and labor. Cooperation among academia, Federal laboratories, labor and industry, in such forms as technology transfer, personnel exchange, joint research projects, and others, should be renewed, expanded, and strengthened.[15]

Similarly, in the 1980 amendments to the patent laws, Congress stated:

It is the policy and objective of the Congress . . . to encourage maximum participation of small business firms in federally supported research and development efforts; to promote collaboration between commercial concerns and nonprofit organizations, including universities; to ensure that inventions made by nonprofit organizations and small business firms are used in a manner to promote free competition and enterprise; to promote the commercialization and public availability of inventions made in the United States by United States industry and labor. . . .[16]

At the same time that it was encouraging academic institutions to establish joint ventures with industry, Congress actively encouraged federal researchers to collaborate with the private sector.[17] Tax incentives continue to encourage investment in research.

The Executive Branch

Earlier this year, the President's Council on Competitiveness recommended that federal agencies "should inform university administrators that seeking commercialization of research in cooperation with U.S. industry is an important element in federally supported university research."[18] This statement echoed ongoing policy of the National Science Foundation (NSF), which has had a program of industry/university cooperative research projects since 1978, according to recent Congressional testimony of Dr. Donald Senich, Director of the NSF Division of Industrial Science and Technological Innovation.[19] The NSF program is designed "to strengthen cooperative science and engineering research on specific problems or issues of mutual interest to university and industrial scientists."[20]

CRITICISMS AND CHALLENGES

Congressional Hearings

Congressional oversight of university/industry relations in biomedical research has included some thoughtful and balanced hearings,[21] as well as hearings focused primarily on alleged abuses.[22] In 1981 and 1982, two subcommittees of the House Committee on Science and Technology (chaired by Albert Gore of Tennessee and Doug Walgren of Pennsylvania) held joint hearings to explore, from a variety of perspectives, the advantages and potential problems inherent in cooperative arrangements between universities and commercial entities.[23] Lead-off witnesses included representatives of Washington University in St. Louis and Monsanto, Co., who described how their collaborative venture was designed to protect academic integrity while infusing the university with the benefits of industrial resources. The important features of the cooperative relationship include: (1) institutional (rather than individual) relationships; (2) faculty-initiated research proposals within broadly defined programs, with faculty participation in selecting the projects to be funded; (3) both internal (faculty) and external (independent) peer review on a regular basis; (4) guaranteed freedom for faculty and students to publish their scientific results; and (5) distribution of financial rewards to the university, academic departments, and individual laboratories responsible for the discoveries (rather than to the responsible faculty members).[24]

As described by Dr. Howard Schneiderman, Monsanto's senior vice president for research and development:

> By combining two of America's greatest resources--the scientific expertise of one of the country's leading medical schools and the technological and scientific capability of a large high technology corporation--we have the opportunity to create new businesses and new jobs, and advance technology. Through this collaboration we expect to discover novel products which address major human diseases and health conditions for which there is presently no cure and no adequate therapy. We view this aim as both socially responsible and commercially attractive.[25]

Congressman Ted Weiss of New York chaired more negative hearings in 1988 and 1989, titled: "Scientific Fraud and Misconduct and the Federal Response";[26] "Federal Response to Misconduct in Science: Are Conflicts of Interest Hazardous to our Health?"[27] and "Is Science For Sale? Conflicts of Interest vs. the Public Interest."[28]

After reviewing several "examples" of the dangers of permitting academic and government scientists to have financial ties to industry, Representative Weiss and his subcommittee concluded in a summary report to Congress that "the Department of HHS should immediately promulgate regulations that clearly restrict financial ties for researchers who conduct evaluations of a product or treatment in which they have a vested interest"; moreover, if the PHS fails to act, "Congress should enact legislation to achieve that goal."[29]

PROPOSED NIH "GUIDELINES"

In response to the congressional investigations, NIH sought to demonstrate that it had matters under control by publishing "guidelines" for academic institutions to follow in dealing with the problem.[30] Many of the provisions in the guidelines seemed to be modeled on the stringent restrictions imposed by Bernadine Healy and her coinvestigators in a multicenter clinical trial of drug administration following coronary artery by-pass surgery.[31] The proposed NIH guidelines would have required, for example, that:

> No investigator, key employee, consultant, or other persons with primary research, management, advisory, supervisory, or purchase authorization responsibilities, or their spouses, dependent children, or other dependents, shall be allowed to have personal equity holdings or options in any company

that would be affected by the outcome of the research or that produces a
product or equipment being evaluated in the research project.[32]

Moreover, "[a]n investigator, key employee, consultant, or other involved
person may not receive honoraria, fees for service, or a management position
from a private source if that individual is involved in an NIH- or ADAMHA-
supported project that is evaluating or testing a product of the source."[33] The
proposed guidelines, however, were drafted with virtually no input from either
the academic community or industry. They were vigorously attacked and quickly
withdrawn, in large part because of a general sense of over-reaching.[34] In
addition, it was correctly observed that the "guidelines" were actually rules of
general applicability and, as such, should be developed as regulations through
the normal rule-making process that affords an opportunity for public comment.

Response to the Proposed Guidelines

In response to the proposed guidelines, some research administrators noted
that existing rules already cover conflicts of interest, while others labeled the
NIH proposal a "bureaucratic nightmare."[35] Karl Hittleman, Associate Vice
Chancellor of the University of California at San Francisco, strongly objected to
the "insidious assumption that seems to underlie the guidelines: that the
university biomedical research community is motivated primarily by venality and
is incapable of self-regulation."[36] Representatives of industry cautioned that the
proposed rules would further erode our country's dominance in biotechnology;
while Robert Weinberg, of the Whitehead Institute, observed: "There are those
in Washington who have the quaint notion that by burying us, quite literally,
under mountains of paperwork, increasingly palpably every year, I and my
colleagues are able to think more clearly and creatively about our science."[37]

Finally, Brook Byers, a venture capitalist, called it a "cruel irony" that the
proposal came "at a time when Congress, the Administration, and the public are
pushing for a closer cooperation between the NIH, academic research, and
companies."[38]

Meanwhile, the American Medical Association, the Association of American Medical Colleges, the Association of Academic Health Centers, and the
Institute of Medicine analyzed the problems inherent in academic/industry
collaborations, described the benefits and the risks to all concerned, and
proposed general guidelines for identifying and dealing with problem situations.[39] Mandatory disclosure of any financial interests of academic faculty in
commercial entities played a central role in all four publications, as did the need
to recognize (and accommodate) the heterogeneity of academic institutions. But
there was no clear delineation of the financial interests or relationships that
should be prohibited across the board, as distinguished from those that might be
acceptable with appropriate disclosure and careful supervision. Those lines
were to be drawn by the individual universities.

THE PUBLIC HEALTH SERVICE TRIES AGAIN

On 30 November 1990, the Public Health Service (PHS) held an "open meeting" at NIH to which representatives from both industry and academe were invited to discuss issues involved in the continuing effort to develop PHS regulations governing "Conflicts of Interest In Clinical Evaluation of Commercial Products."[40] In announcing the meeting, the PHS indicated that "the overarching issue is how best to protect the integrity of research while promoting technology transfer," consistent with the following general principles:

- Efficient transfer of research results into commerce is and will continue to be essential if the US is to maintain and enhance health-care and economic competitiveness.
- Pertinent federal statutes provide generally that tax-financed research institutions will give high priority to ensuring commercialization of their scientists' results wherever appropriate.
- The research community will not maintain public confidence without rules that harmonize the national interest, institutional interest, and individual interests.
- There is an apparent need for rules on conflict of interest that will protect the integrity of PHS-sponsored clinical trials and ensure that financial interests of investigators will not compromise the conduct or reporting of such research.
- At the same time, the PHS must strive to ensure that procedures for protection against conflict of interest do not stifle the advancement of research and technology transfer, which are key aspects of the PHS mission.[41]

Since the meeting, a revised proposal has been prepared but, at the time of this writing, it is undergoing review by the new NIH Director, Bernadine Healy. An unpublished draft of the proposed rules reveals an absence of specific prohibitions and primary reliance on grantee institutions to devise their own mechanisms and standards to assure that the conduct and reporting of research to evaluate commercial products are not compromised by any financial interests of the research personnel and/or their immediate families. The only absolute requirement in the current draft is that researchers disclose financial interests "that could appreciate or be devalued by the outcome of a PHS-supported clinical trial." It remains to be seen to what extent Dr. Healy's personal views on the subject, reflected in the restrictive guidelines adopted for her coronary artery study,[42] will shape NIH policy. In her confirmation hearings before the Senate, Dr. Healy took a position more supportive of cooperation between academia and industry:

If we are ever to realize the mission of NIH, technology transfer must work. The discoveries of the laboratory must be carried to the bedside, and the development of new drugs, devices, and diagnostic tests needs to be done in partnership with industry. The Federal government has developed a strong legislative portfolio over the past decade to foster that transfer. As in any new venture, the implementation has uncovered some real or perceived problems with the partnerships and their incentives. But those difficulties are not a reason to walk away from a principle of great social value; they provide an impetus to develop carefully crafted guidelines to help industry, academia and government work together for the right reasons and not be tarnished by even a hint of wrong ones.[43]

It is difficult to quarrel with that statement. The ultimate challenge is to translate it into practice, and to convince Congress that further legislation is not required.

CONCLUSION

Proposed PHS regulations are likely to be published for public comment within the next few months. In my view, any rule making in this area should include:

- Uniform definitions and standards applicable government-wide, to all federally funded biomedical research;
- Flexibility for institutions to adopt those standards to their existing governance structure and individual needs;
- Primary reliance on grantee institutions to implement and monitor compliance with the standards;
- Avoidance of retroactive application of the definitions and standards.

Rather than pressing for prompt rule making, it would be better to establish a deliberative body (much like the National Commission for the Protection of Human Subjects) with members representing diverse interests and expertise (for example, university faculty, administrators, and counsel; industrial sponsors; federal agency officials; representatives of the general public; and others experienced in law and public policy). Such a panel could conduct all of its hearings and deliberations in public and permit unlimited access to all materials under consideration, thus affording affected parties as much participation as possible in the deliberative process. That is the best method of achieving a reasonable accommodation of legitimate interests that appear to be in conflict, and it will enhance public confidence in both the process and the resulting guidelines (which then could be promulgated as regulations).

NOTES

1   Association of Academic Health Centers (AAHC), Task Force on Science Policy, *Conflicts of Interest in Academic Health Centers* (Washington, DC: AAHC, 1990); Institute of Medicine, *Government and Industry Collaboration in Biomedical Research and Education* (Washington, DC: National Academy Press, 1989); D. Nelkin, R. Nelson, and C. Kiernan, "Commentary: University-Industry Alliances," *Science, Technology, and Human Values* 12 (1987):65-74.

2   Nelkin, Nelson, and Kiernan, "Commentary"; Morrill Act (Act of 2 July 1862), ch. 30, codified at 7 USC, sec. 301 *et seq.*

3   Morrill Act.

4   AAHC, *Conflicts of Interest*; Institute of Medicine, *Government and Industry Collaboration*.

5   AAHC, *Conflicts of Interest*.

6   Institute of Medicine, *Government and Industry Collaboration*.

7   A. Hayes, "Statement announcing FDA approval of hepatitis B vaccine," *HHS News* (16 November 1981), reprinted in US House of Representatives, Committee on Science and Technology, *Hearings on University/Industry Cooperation in Biotechnology*, 16-17 June 1982 (Washington, DC: US Government Printing Office, 1982).

8   President's Council on Competitiveness, *Report on National Biotechnology Policy* (Washington, DC: Department of Commerce, 1991).

9   *Ibid.*

10   Committee on Science and Technology, *Hearings*.

11   AAHC, *Conflicts of Interest*; Institute of Medicine, *Government and Industry Collaboration*; American Medical Association, Council on Scientific Affairs and Council on Ethical and Judicial Affairs, "Conflicts of Interest in Medical Center/Industry Research Relationships," *Journal of the American Medical Association* 263 (1990):2790-93; B. Healy, L. Campeau, R. Gray, *et al.*, "Conflict of Interest Guidelines for a Multicenter Clinical Trial after Coronary-Artery Bypass-Grant Surgery," *New England Journal of Medicine* 320 (1989):949-51.

12   AAHC, *Conflicts of Interest*; Institute of Medicine, *Government and Industry Collaboration*; President's Council on Competitiveness, *Report.*

13   AAHC, *Conflicts of Interest*; American Medical Association, "Conflicts of Interest"; Association of American Medical Colleges, *Guidelines for Dealing With Faculty Conflicts of Commitment and Conflicts of Interest in Research* (Washington, DC: AAMC, 1990).

14   Stevenson-Wydler Technology Innovation Act of 1980, Pub. L. 96-480, 5 USC, sec. 370(3), 3702(5).

15   *Ibid.*

16   Patent and Trademark Amendments Act of 1980, Pub. L. 96517, 35 USC, sec. 200 (1988).

17   Federal Technology Transfer Act of 1986, Pub. L. 99-502, 5 USC, sec. 3710.
18   President's Council on Competitiveness, *Report.*
19   Committee on Science and Technology, *Hearings.*
20   *Ibid.*
21   *Ibid.*
22   US House of Representatives, Committee on Energy and Commerce, Subcommittee on Oversight and Investigations, *Hearings on Scientific Fraud* (Washington, DC: US Government Printing Office, 30 April and 14 May 1990); US House of Representatives, Committee on Government Operations, *Are Scientific Misconduct and Conflicts of Interest Hazardous to our Health?* (Washington, DC: US Government Printing Office, 1990).
23   Committee on Science and Technology, *Hearings.*
24   US House of Representatives, Committee on Government Operations, Subcommittee on Human Resources and Intergovernmental Relations *Hearing on Scientific Fraud and Misconduct and the Federal Response,* (Washington DC: US Government Printing Office, 1988).
25   Committee on Science and Technology, *Hearings.*
26   Committee of Government Operations, *Hearing on Scientific Fraud.*
27   US House of Representatives, Committee on Government Operations, Subcommittee on Human Resources and Intergovernmental Relations, *Federal Response to Misconduct in Science: Are Conflicts of Interest Hazardous to Our Health?* (Washington, DC: US Government Printing Office, 1988).
28   US House of Representatives, Committee on Government Operations, Subcommittee on Human Resources and Intergovernmental Relations, *Is Science for Sale? Conflicts of Interest vs. the Public Interest* (Washington, DC: US Government Printing Office, 1989).
29   Committee on Government Operations, *Are Scientific Misconduct and Conflicts of Interest Hazardous?*
30   US Department of Health and Human Services, *NIH Guide for Grants and Contracts* 18, no.2 (1989).
31   Healy, Campeau, Gray, *et al.,* "Conflict of Interest."
32   US Department of Health and Human Services, *NIH Guide.*
33   *Ibid.* ADAMHA is the Alcohol, Drug Abuse, and Mental Health Administration.
34   J. Palca, "NIH Conflict of Interest Guidelines Shot Down," *Science* 247 (1990):153-56.
35   J. Palca, "Some of the Voices from the Chorus of Protest," *Science* 247 (1990):155.
36   *Ibid.*
37   *Ibid.*
38   *Ibid.*
39   AAHC, *Conflicts of Interest;* Institute of Medicine, *Government and Industry*

Collaboration; American Medical Association, "Conflicts of Interest"; Association of American Medical Colleges, *Guidelines*.

40 US Department of Health and Human Services, Public Health Service, Open Meeting on Conflicts of Interest in Clinical Evaluation of Commercial Products, *Federal Register* 55 (1990):45815-16.

41 *Ibid*.

42 Healy, Campeau, Gray, *et al.*, "Conflict of Interest."

43 B. Healy, "Statement Before the Senate Committee on Labor and Human Resources," reprinted in *The NIH Record* (2 April 1991):1, 6-7.

17

Role of Conflict of Interest in Public Advisory Councils

Adil E. Shamoo

Nowadays, it is taken as an article of faith that "advisory groups" render objective and unbiased opinions regarding important public-health policy issues and the relative worth of projects for funding. These "advisory groups" include advisory councils, advisory boards, study sections, review panels, and various other names. The US government uses these advisory groups widely; they are relied upon extensively for policy decisions that affect issues relevant to public health and public expenditure of billions of dollars, ranging from drugs to environmental concerns. The heavy reliance on such groups is primarily based on two premises: (1) expertise in the subject area and (2) objectivity. The public-health services (Department of Health and Human Services), with its various components such as the National Institutes of Health (NIH) and Alcohol, Drug Abuse, and Mental Health Administration (ADAMHA), represent one of the largest government agencies that rely heavily on the advisory opinions of these groups. NIH and ADAMHA represent practically all of the activities of the public-health services with regard to the topic of this paper. The issue we would like to address here is the "objectivity" of the members of these advisory councils. Koshland stated in his *Science* magazine editorial that "Modern

Data for this investigation came as a result of inquiry to Office of Scientific Integrity Review (OSIR), US Public Health Service, Department of Health and Human Services, and were provided by Dr. William E. McGarvey, Statistical Analysis Unit; Statistics, Analysis, and Evaluation Section; Information Systems Branch; Division of Research Grants; NIH; Bethesda, MD 20892.

The author wishes to thank Dr. Marie Cassidy of George Washington University and Dr. Leslie J. Glick of Bionix Corp. for their valuable comments on the manuscript. Many thanks to Ms. Cheryl Douglass for editing the manuscript.

specialization makes it inevitable that those who evaluate complex subjects must have the relevant expertise within that profession to make fair judgments."[1] Concern and suspicions regarding the "objectivity" of these "boards" have been expressed as early as these boards were utilized.[2] It is for this reason that the term "old boy network" was coined.[3]

The use of different forms of "peer review" expanded during this century.[4] It appears that the development of peer review for funding of projects, or establishing public policy, was parallel to that for publication. The grant peer-review process was established by law in 1937, for grants from the National Cancer Institute.[5] Since then, numerous laws and statutes have been enacted, empowering various bodies as peer-review boards. Burnham's conclusion was that the peer-review process was institutionalized in order "to meet demands for expert authority and objectivity in an increasingly specialized world."[6]

In modern legal ethics literature,[7] the issue of avoidance of conflict of interest, or the appearance of conflict of interest, by judges and lawyers is extensively addressed to ensure that the legal system incorporates the values of fairness and integrity. This issue is even more extensively addressed in the financial literature so as to provide detailed methods of avoidance of conflict of interest, and to provide in a periodic fashion independent sources of judgment on various financial transactions.[8] In the health-care delivery field, there are ample precedents and laws to enhance an independent judgment by peers who are usually not direct competitors for the same sources of reward.[9] It is ironic that, virtually in science alone, direct competitors--and not independent judgments--are used as "advisory groups" for their "objective" opinion. In every subfield of science, the group's number may be a few dozen, of which literally everyone knows each other. This personal and professional knowledge of one another, coupled with the fact that most of the members of each group are direct competitors, would seem to render these members of advisory groups incapable of truly impartial and objective opinions. This situation has arisen for several reasons, including (1) the limited number of trained professionals in this arena; (2) their degree of specialization; and (3) consequently, an element of elitism.

In this article, we are not addressing the issue of financial conflict of interests that may face advisory groups. There have been several reports on this issue, including a detailed report by the Human Resources and Intergovernmental Relations Subcommittee of the US Congress, chaired by Congressman Ted Weiss.[10]

Usually, members of the advisory councils are experts in their field and thus play dual roles as direct competitors for, and recipients of, public funding from the same government agency. Members of the councils have a very large influence, not only on the funding of a specific project, but also on the overall direction of the research endeavor of that particular agency or its component. These "experts" tend to develop strong personal relationships with the staff of the agency, who exert considerable influence on the selection of experts and, more importantly, on the overall research thrust. The purpose of these "advisory groups" is to exercise a certain degree of control over the quality of the projects and policies, and to facilitate the development of products and services to the public.[11] Problems in this system may arise from two sources: (1) conflict between the desire for quality data and facilitation of innovation; and (2) the interests of those sitting in judgment of these projects.

In the recent past, we have proposed a way to improve and control quality of data by auditing the data that are intended as the basis for products, services, or public policy.[12] At the same time, under the heading "Creative Process and Data Audit," we have vigorously defended the rights of the investigator to be protected from outside interference that could stifle creativity during the initial discovery period of the investigation.[13] As a matter of fact, we even argued that these initial discovery periods should not be subject to any audit. The second source of problems is the conflict of interest. We have addressed this issue and its avoidance in detail elsewhere.[14]

Many believe that complete avoidance of conflict of interest in the advisory boards can only be accomplished by lowering the caliber of "expertise" available. Conversely, however, is the belief that the caliber of innovation may be significantly enhanced since censorship due to conflict of interest and bias would be greatly reduced. Experts can continue to provide "technical reviews" if needed; they need not to be responsible for the ultimate decision. However, when 10 to 15 percent of approved grants proposed are funded, the whole selection process of meritorious projects become extremely cloudy. (We take for granted that censorship in a modern civilized society is anathema, and that it violates basic human rights). Even though advisory groups do not intentionally exercise censorship, these groups tend to be conservative (that is, allied with doctrinal concepts) by design, and thus are very likely to be inhospitable to unpopular or new projects.

Hillman has recently published a paper entitled "Resistance to the Spread of Unpopular Academic Findings and Views in Liberal Societies, including a Personal Case."[15] The article chronicles current mechanisms that prevent unpopular research from being funded and communicated. Moreover, the author points out the danger to our society from such censorship of ideas and research. Horrobin lists dozens of cases of innovative, truly breakthrough works that were either censored, hampered, or misdirected by the peer-review process.[16] In reference to risk management, Greenberg et al. have coined the term "Biased Objectivity Oxymoron" to describe the type of dilemma faced by panel members.[17]

Unfortunately, the analysis of public policy, which includes the influence of bias and many other various parameters, cannot be easily quantified. Therefore, the topic does not lend itself to simple scientific analysis. Despite these difficulties, we would like to address this complex issue. In this approach, we will attempt to meld together the quantifiable and the nonquantifiable approaches. Public policies regarding research have the greatest influence on the integrity of science.

The particular question addressed in this chapter is whether membership in these advisory groups gives its members, and thus their projects, most favored treatment in receiving funding from these agencies. We should keep in mind that this particular question is selected to serve as an illustrative example rather than a comprehensive treatment. The underlying hypothesis is that council members enjoy advantages during, and after, their service on such review panels. To address this question, records were culled from the PHS's Open/Pending, History, Committee Management, and Appointment files for the years 1979 through 1989. Using all new and competing grants in the public health service, and different types of grants such as Type 1, R01, P01.... and so on, four different membership status levels were defined: (1) Prior Members; (2) Current Members; (3) Later Members; and (4) Non-Members. Please note that Type 1 represents new grant applications. Types 2 and 9 represent competing renewals.

METHODS

We have utilized the following two sources of information:

1. A public document entitled "DRG, Peer Review Trends--Members Characteristics: DRG Study Section, Institute Review Groups, Advisory Councils and Boards, 1977-1986," published by Information Systems Branch, Division of Research Grants, National Institutes of Health. The data, figures, and tables were taken directly from this booklet.
2. Data were obtained as a result of a request made by the author to the Office of Scientific Integrity Review, and were provided by Dr. William E. McGarvey of NIH.[18]

Records were culled from the Open/Pending, History, Committee Management, and Appointment Files for the Years 1979 through 1989. Using only new, or Type 1 R01 grant applications, and P grant applications[19] four different membership status levels were defined: (1) Prior Members--those scientists who had council appointment and termination dates for council service that preceded the fiscal year of the initial review group (IRG) review of their application; (2) Current Members--scientists whose council appointment date for council service preceded the fiscal year of IRG review of their application and whose termination date followed such review; (3) Later Members--scientists whose applications were reviewed before their council service dates; and (4) Non-Members--scientists who submitted applications, but never served on a council.

RESULTS AND DISCUSSION

Composition of "Advisory Groups"

Advisory councils at the institute level are the only ones that contain non-scientists. In the context of this chapter, only the scientific members of the "advisory groups" are considered. In contrast, study sections more accurately represent the "experts" and, hopefully, all members of each subdiscipline. Study sections are several steps lower in hierarchy than advisory councils. The higher level advisory groups within Public Health Service are medical degree holders; therefore, the composition of advisory councils often does not coincide with training in the discipline. Close to 58 percent of the members of advisory councils hold MD degrees, whereas only 33.2 percent of study sections have MD degrees.[20]

Study Sections

Figure 17.1 shows data on mean priority scores of current study section members versus other R01 applicants, for October 1977 through 1986. R01 applications are investigator-initiated research grant proposals. The data show that for both types of applications, the mean priority score for members of the study section are well below those of non-members. It should be emphasized here that a lower score in this system translates into a greater likelihood of funding, a type of ranking oxymoron. This is even more dramatically illustrated in Figure 17.2, where success rates of current and former study section members are compared to other research grant applicants. The data show that members of study sections are much more successful in grant awards than non-members. However, a closer look at the mean scores before, during, and after serving in study sections indicates that there may be a statistical advantage after such service, and only with respect to new R01 applications. These differences may be due to several factors, such as members of study sections have better scientific skills (this would be consistent with the use of the word "experts"); (2) members receive "favored treatment"; and (3) members become more knowledgeable about the system and use it to their advantage.

As I have mentioned earlier, public-policy issues do not always lend themselves to neat clear-cut statistical analysis. Nevertheless, we can propose that these constant differences may be due to one or more factors. The most reasonable projection is that it is due to a combination of all these factors, with factor 3 alone being the most likely to favor the outcome of their own efforts.

Advisory Councils

Table 17.1 gives the statistical data on the Public Health Services competing R01 grants for prior, current, later members, and non-members of PHS advisory councils. Figure 17.3 is a plot of these data. Based upon a frequency-weighted

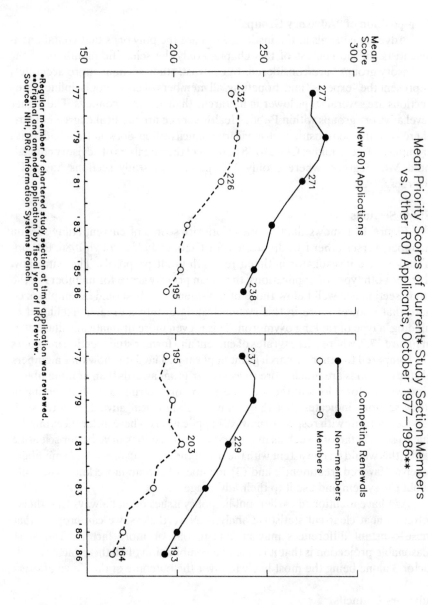

Fig. 17.1.

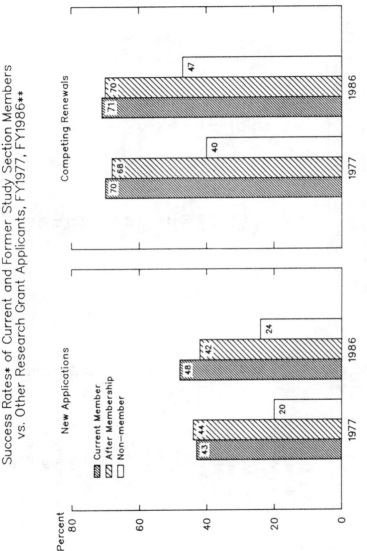

Fig. 17.2.

TABLE 17.1

Statistics on PHS Competing R01 Grants for Prior, Current, and Later Members of PHS Advisory Councils, Type 1

FISCAL YEAR OF IRG	REVIEW STATUS	NUMBER OF MEMBERS	NUMBER REVIEWED	NUMBER APPROVED	AVERAGE NUMBER AWARDED	MEDIAN APPROVED SCORE	APPROVED SCORE
1979	Prior Member	17	20	15	5	306.5	344.0
	Current Member	12	13	12	8	222.4	193.5
	Later Member	53	69	51	22	256.5	237.0
	Non-Member	10,951	13,107	8,606	3,467	275.8	266.0
1980	Prior Member	26	31	22	13	238.0	209.5
	Current Member	12	12	9	5	227.0	212.0
	Later Member	42	54	40	21	240.2	235.0
	Non-Member	10,662	12,596	8,419	2,829	272.3	264.0
1981	Prior Member	15	15	10	4	234.7	250.0
	Current Member	15	17	12	7	245.0	223.5
	Later Member	45	56	40	20	235.8	210.0
	Non-Member	10,557	12,590	8,883	2,496	265.5	256.0
1982	Prior Member	20	21	19	11	209.4	185.0
	Current Member	7	8	6	1	263.0	258.5
	Later Member	38	47	37	21	203.4	190.0
	Non-Member	10,332	12,457	9,295	2,461	256.8	247.0
1983	Prior Member	20	23	21	4	243.2	228.0
	Current Member	11	14	11	3	253.8	251.0
	Later Member	34	39	29	15	211.7	199.0
	Non-Member	10,646	12,735	9,916	2,889	248.6	240.0

Table 17.1 continued next page

Table 17.1.

Fiscal Year of IRG Review	Status	Number of Members	Number Reviewed	Number Approved	Average Number Awarded	Median Approved Score	Approved Score
1984	Prior Member	29	36	31	8	226.3	229.0
	Current Member	11	16	11	5	263.8	238.0
	Later Member	27	33	31	17	200.3	178.0
	Non-Member	11,038	13,301	10,674	3,037	245.2	234.0
1985	Prior Member	29	32	30	7	234.8	234.5
	Current Member	10	11	9	6	213.6	176.0
	Later Member	29	34	32	15	195.4	181.5
	Non-Member	11,601	14,310	11,882	3,096	239.7	228.0
1986	Prior Member	17	23	21	4	239.8	220.0
	Current Member	8	10	10	6	198.9	165.5
	Later Member	17	24	18	6	233.2	209.5
	Non-Member	10,539	12,764	10,741	2,770	234.7	221.0
1987	Prior Member	26	30	28	10	233.8	202.5
	Current Member	16	24	19	7	197.2	201.0
	Later Member	16	18	16	10	199.8	150.0
	Non-Member	10,251	12,452	10,480	2,811	236.1	221.0
1988	Prior Member	22	22	20	6	243.1	195.5
	Current Member	20	29	26	11	227.6	224.0
	Later Member	11	12	11	8	173.4	148.0
	Non-Member	10,417	12,456	10,923	2,429	246.4	233.0
1989	Prior Member	30	33	32	6	268.6	247.5
	Current Member	12	14	13	7	206.8	188.0
	Later Member	6	6	5	1	166.0	263.0
	Non-Member	11,447	14,105	13,115	2,471	259.4	248.0

Note: All fiscal years of IRG Review include January, May, and October Council Rounds. Source: Open/Pending, History, Committee Management and Appointment Files. NIH/DRG/ISB/SAES/SAU/WEM

Median Priority Scores for Approved R01 Applications of Prior, Current, Later, and Non-Members of NIH Councils, FY 1979-1989

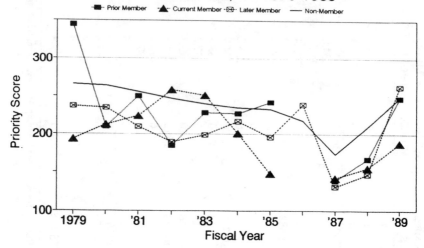

N.B. All fiscal years of IRG Review include January, May, and October Council Rounds. As there were only two prior and two current members who submitted proposals in 1986, these points have been omitted. Source: Open/Pending, History, Committee Management and Appointment Files. NIH/DRG/ISB/SAES/SAU/WEM

Fig. 17.3

average priority score across the entire time period, later members enjoy the greatest relative advantage (mean = 225.6), followed by current members (mean = 230.3), prior members (mean = 244.2), and then non-members (mean = 255.3). As the figure suggests, though, the disparity seems most pronounced since 1987; both means and medians over the period 1979 through 1985 were volatile in their relative ordering. These differences are relatively small and may simply reflect several factors mentioned earlier, including the "quality" and "expert" nature of these members.

The most interesting data are shown in Table 17.2. An award, of course, is the ultimate initial aim of the grant application. Table 17.2 shows the number of approved and awarded Type 1 (new) R01 applications of non-members, compared to members of PHS Advisory Councils, FY 1979 through 1989. It is clear that non-members face stiff competition among their peers, since approved grants are awarded to only 27.2 percent. Indeed, the applications from prior ($p < 0.005$), current ($p < 0.005$), and later members ($p < 0.005$) of the council enjoy far greater probability of funding (50.3 to 35.9 percent) than non-members (almost twice as much in the case of current members). These differences are even more astonishing in light of the fact that priority score differentials are rather modest. This strong conclusion is further augmented by the fact that the data are restricted to new applications, which are supposed to be truly competitive as compared to competing renewals. Funding of a grant application depends on several factors; these include the priority scores or, more recently, percentile score. Other factors are programmatic in nature; and thus, each program in a designated institute may have a different cut-off point. Council members could have the greatest influence on assigning their application into a specific program. Also, inside knowledge of an institute's "research portfolio" could further enhance their funding prospects.

TABLE 17.2

Number of Approved and Awarded Type 1 (New) R01 Applications of Members of PHS Advisory Councils, FY 1979-1989

STATUS OF COUNCIL MEMBER	NUMBER APPROVED	NUMBER AWARDED	PERCENT AWARDED	P VALUE
Prior Member	217	78	35.9	$p < .005$
Current Member	138	66	47.8	$p < .005$
Later Member	310	156	50.3	$p < .005$
Non-Member	112,934	30,756	27.2	

Note: Data derived from Table 1 (see Methods section for details). The *p* values are derived from Chi Square, comparing each row with non-members.

There are several kinds of research program projects and center grants awarded by PHS to applicant organizations. For example, P01, Research Program Projects; P20, Exploratory Grants; P30, Center Core Grants, and others as defined by IMPAC booklet.[21] These types of grant applications are not open to everyone, as is the case in R01 applications. These applications are usually only initiated following intense consultation with relevant institute staff. Therefore, there exists a preselection process by which advisory council members can exert an influence. Figure 17.4 shows that data on median priority scores for approved P applications for council members and non-members FY 1979 through 1989. There are no significant statistical differences in the priority scores. Table 17.3 presents the data on the number of approved and awarded P applications Types 1,2, and 9 (new and competing renewals) of members of PHS advisory councils, FY 1979 through 1989. The table shows that, in general, those who are non-members of the council (but are already a selected group) have a 56.3 percent chance of being awarded, while investigators in the other designated categories

Median Priority Scores for Approved P Applications of Prior, Current, Later, and Non-Members of PHS Councils, FY 1979-1989

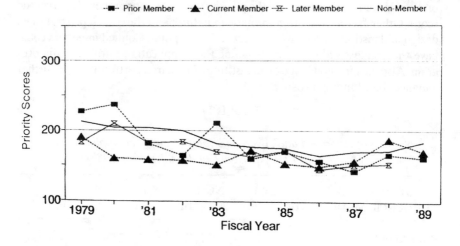

N.B. All fiscal years of IRG Review include January, May, and October Council Rounds.
Source: Open/Pending, History, Committee Management and Appointment Files. NIH/DRG/ISB/SAES/SAU/WEM

Fig. 17.4

TABLE 17.3

Number of Approved and Awarded Types 1, 2, and 9 (New and Competing Renewal) P Applications of Members of PHS Advisory Councils, FY 1979-1989

STATUS OF COUNCIL MEMBER	NUMBER APPROVED	NUMBER AWARDED	PERCENT AWARDED	*P* VALUE
Prior Member	122	80	65.6	$p < .05$
Current Member	79	59	74.7	$p < .005$
Later Member	143	113	79.0	$p < .001$
Non-Member	5,110	2,879	56.3	

Note: The *p* values are derived from Chi Square, comparing each row with Non-Members.

are much higher, up to 79 percent (again, p ranging from less than 0.05 to 0.001, when non-members were compared to either current members or later members). These numbers show that the review process plays a minor role in the final awarding of the research funds, since the ratio of awardee to applicants is so high. New and competing renewal grant applications are supposed to be similarly treated during the review process. Table 17.4 presents the data on the number of approved and awarded P applications Types 1 (new) only. The table shows that, in general again, those who are non-members of the council (but are already a selected group) have a 42.7 percent chance of being awarded, while investigators in the other designated categories are much higher, up to 61.5 percent. Only later members (61.5 percent) show statistical significance from non-members (42.7 percent). The lack of statistical significance for the other two categories reflects the fact that we are dealing with small numbers when we restricted the data for new grants only.

TABLE 17.4

Number of Approved and Awarded Type 1 (New) P Applications of Members of PHS Advisory Councils, FY 1979-1989

STATUS OF COUNCIL MEMBER	NUMBER APPROVED	NUMBER AWARDED	PERCENT AWARDED	P VALUE
Prior Member	50	24	48.0	$p > .1$
Current Member	29	17	58.6	$p > .1$
Later Member	52	32	61.5	$p > .01$
Non-Member	2,769	1,183	42.7	

Note: The p values are derived from Chi Square, comparing each row with non-members.

In an attempt to determine the percent of members of the councils who receive P-type grants, we made the following assumptions. For the FY 1979 through 1989, the council membership turnover is 2.5 times (four-year terms); there are about ten scientists in each council; and there are fifteen relevant institutes. This will give us 375 council members (a high estimate). From Table 17.3, there are 252 awards during the same period for council members. Therefore 67 percent of council members receive P-type grants (not counting R01s). The high percentage of members of councils with potentially vested financial interest could adversely affect the "objectivity" of these members in determining the funding and direction of research programs.

In an official NIH cover letter, transmitted with the data to this author, signed by Dr. McGarvey and cleared by NIH officials, Dr. McGarvey states:

While the data may suggest that Members do enjoy some advantage over Non-Members, there are a couple of points that deserve repeating. Firstly, as the ordering of frequency-weighted R01 priority scores suggests, it is Later Members or Current Members--not Prior Members--who may be doing better. This advantage may arise for a variety of possible reasons, not involving any conflict of interest. Secondly, any discussion of PHS Council Members is inevitably a small, numerically limited set of cases, and inferences should be appropriately restrained. Thirdly, these data bear upon all of PHS, and are not limited to only NIH.[22]

The author of this article stands by his conclusions.

CONCLUSIONS

Wolfram, in discussing conflicts of interest in the legal profession, states: "Its importance, as well as its difficulty, is that conflicts of interest are part of the world around us, always have been, and inevitably must be."[23]

This is obviously true for the science profession also. Wolfram continues when he describes lawyers: "They are human beings of the same general sort as the rest of humanity, with their own interests, their own hopes and aspirations, their own bank accounts and investments, their own nagging pressures of personal belief and personal life."

This description could have been written for scientists or any other professional group. However, because of these multiple masters and interests, awareness and avoidance of conflict of interest should be exercised for the better good of the public. Conflict of interest may be manifested at any level, from the individual to the agency. This was discussed, for example, by Boruch and George in detailing the conflict arising from government agencies that deal both with enforcement and with research.[24] With respect to these two missions, there is a host of conflict interests that must be acknowledged and dealt with in order to maintain the public's confidence in the agency. In reference to publication bias, Chalmers et al. suggest that peer reviewers and authors be required to acknowledge conflicts of interest.[25] McNutt et al. found that blinding improves the quality of peer review.[26]

Cantekin et al. in discussing their own case states: "The current peer review system as shown by this case, is unable to embrace dissent within the peer review process and to use dissent to serve scientific truth and the public interest."[27]

Koshland stated: "There has to be a reasonable compromise between expertise and conflict."[28]

However, a reasonable compromise could be reached by designing decision-making structures that either avoid or minimize the conflict of interest. The current advisory group composition and structure appears to have neither avoided nor minimized conflict of interest. It is in this spirit that we propose that advisory groups should have the following characteristics:

1. They should reflect the profession's composition (that is, PhDs, MDs, engineers, and so on). We should provide no specific quota.
2. Direct competitors should not serve on advisory groups. They could serve on other advisory groups where their expertise is not in direct competition with other applicants projects. If "direct competitors" are absolutely needed, then "technical advice" can be attained without a decision-making or voting power.
3. If direct competitors with conflicting interests are absolutely needed to serve in a given advisory group, then their percentage should not exceed 20 percent. Moreover, their conflict of interest should be clearly stated.
4. The deliberation of "advice" should be open and a quick "rebuttal" should be a part of the deliberation prior to voting merit scores.

NOTES

1   D.E. Koshland, "Conflict of Interest," *Science* 249 (1990):109.

2   K. Dickersin, "The Existence of Publication Bias and Risk Factors for its Occurrence," *Journal of the American Medical Association* 263 (1990):1385-89; J.C. Burnham, "The Evolution of Editorial Peer Review," *Journal of the American Medical Association* 263 (1990):1323-29.

3   Burnham, "Evolution of Editorial Peer Review."

4   *Ibid.*

5   Dickersin, "Existence of Publication Bias."

6   Burnham, "Evolution of Editorial Peer Review."

7   C.W. Wolfram, *Modern Legal Ethics* (St. Paul, MN: West Publishing, 1986).

8   American Institute of Certified Public Accountants (AICPA) Statement on Standards for Attestation Engagements, "Attestation Standards," (New York: AICPA, 1986); S.E. Loeb and A.E. Shamoo, "Data Audit: Its Place in Auditing," *Accountability in Research* 1 (1989):23-32.

9   A. Donabedian, "Evaluating the Quality of Medical Care," *Milbank Memorial Quarterly* 402 (1966):166-206; M.S. Donaldson and K. Keith, "Planning for Program Effectiveness in Quality Assurance," in *Evaluation and the Health Profession* 6 (1983): 233-44.

10 Committee on Government Operations, "Are Scientific Misconduct and Conflict of Interest Hazardous to Our Health?" US House Report No. 101-688, *Nineteenth Report* (1990):1-74.

11 D.F. Horrobin, "The Philosophical Basis of Peer Review and the Suppression of Innovation," *Journal of the American Medical Association* 263 (1990):1438-41.

12   A.E. Shamoo and S. Davis, "The Need for Integration of Data Audit into Research and Development Operations," in *Principles of Research Data Audit,* ed. A.E. Shamoo (New York: Gordon and Breach Science Publishers, 1989), 27-38.

13   A.E. Shamoo and Z. Annau, "Data Audit--Historical Perspective," in *Principles of Research Data Audit,* 1-11.

14   Shamoo and Davis, "The Need for Integration."

15   H. Hillman, "Resistance to the Spread of Unpopular Academic Findings and Views in Liberal Societies, Including a Personal Case," *Accountability in Research* 1 (1991):259-72.

16   Horrobin, "The Philosophical Basis."

17   M.R. Greenberg, H. Spiro, and R. McIntyre, "Ethical Oxymora for Risk Assessment Practicers," *Accountability in Research* 1 (1991):245-58.

18   William E. McGarvey, MD, of the Statistical Analysis Unit; Statistics, Analysis, and Evaluation Section; Information Systems Branch; Division of Research Grants; NIH, Bethesda, MD 20892; letter to the authors.

19   Shamoo and Davis, "The Need for Integration."

20   IMPAC, "Activity Codes, Organization Codes, and Definitions Used in Extramural Programs: A Computer-Based Information System of the Extramural Programs at NIH/PHS," (Bethesda, MD: NIH, Division of Research Grants, Information Systems Branch, February 1991).

21   *Ibid.*

22   McGarvey, letter to the authors.

23   Wolfram, *Modern Legal Ethics.*

24   R.S. Barouch and V. George, "Mitigating Ethical Conflicts in Dual Mission Government Agencies," *Science, Technology, and Human Values* 13 (1988):27-44.

25   T.C. Chalmers, C.S. Frank, and D. Reitman, "Minimizing The three Stages of Publication Bias," *Journal of the American Medical Association* 263 (1990):1392-95.

26   R.A. McNutt, A.T. Evans, R.H. Fletcher, and S.W. Fletcher, "The Effects of Blinding on the Quality of Peer Review," *Journal of the American Medical Association* 263 (1990):1371-76.

27   E.I. Cantekin, T.W. McGuire, and R.L. Potter, "Biomedical Information, Peer Review, and Conflict of Interest as they Influence Public Health," *Journal of the American Medical Association* 263 (1990):1427-30.

28   Koshland, "Conflict of Interest."

Part III

Scientific Response to External Pressures: Research on Human Subjects

18

International Ethical Considerations for Research on Human Subjects

Zbigniew Bankowski

So act as to treat humanity, whether in thine own person or in that of any other in every case as an end and, withal, never as a means only.

Immanuel Kant

Advances in the biomedical sciences and in medical technology, and their application in the practice of medicine, are provoking some anxiety among the public and confronting society with new ethical dilemmas. Society is expressing its concern about what it fears would be abuses in scientific investigation and biomedical technology.

This concern is understandable in view of the methods of biomedical experimental research and their application. Investigation begins with the construction of hypotheses that are tested in laboratories and with experimental animals. For the findings to be clinically useful, experiments must be performed on human subjects and, even though carefully designed, such research entails some risk to the subjects. This risk is justified not by any personal benefit to the researcher or the research institution, but rather by its benefit to the human subjects involved, and its potential contribution to human knowledge--to the relief of suffering or to the prolongation of life. Long-term benefits are likely to be collective.

Society, together with the medical profession, devises measures to protect against possible abuses. Thus, after the Second World War, the judgments passed by the Nuremberg Tribunal on those who ran the Nazi concentration

This paper is based largely on material contributed to the Council for International Organizations of Medical Sciences conferences on health policy, ethics, and human values.

camps laid down the standards for carrying out human experimentation, emphasizing the subject's voluntary consent. Later, the medical profession, represented by the World Medical Association, took an important step to further reassure society: it adopted the Helsinki Declaration of 1964. This declaration was elaborated and revised in 1975, and again in 1983 and 1989; it provides ethical guidelines for research involving human subjects.

In view of the special circumstances of developing countries with regard to the applicability of the Nuremberg Code and the Declaration of Helsinki, the Council for International Organizations of Medical Sciences (CIOMS) and the World Health Organization (WHO) undertook in the late 1970s a further examination of these matters. In 1982, the organizations issued their Proposed International Guidelines for Biomedical Research Involving Human Subjects.

Ethicists, medical practitioners, and biomedical research workers agree that health-care practice and all biomedical research involving human subjects should be conducted in accordance with the general principles of ethics; namely, *respect for persons, beneficence,* and *justice.* In the United States, these principles were formulated by the National Commission for the Protection of Human Subjects of Biomedical and Behavioural Research and published in 1978 in the Belmont Report. They are generally considered to be the ultimate foundation for any further, second-order principles, rules, and norms. Both the Declaration of Helsinki and the WHO/CIOMS Guidelines uphold and embody these ethical principles, and they provide guidance regarding their application in specific contexts.

Respect for persons is a general principle that incorporates two further principles: *autonomy* and *protection of those with impaired or diminished autonomy.* The principle of autonomy requires that people who are capable of deliberation about their personal goals, and of acting under the direction of their conclusions, be treated with respect for their self-determination. The principle of autonomy requires that adequate information be given to those invited to join studies as subjects, and that they are told the truth regarding such studies. The principle applies to individuals, groups, and communities intended to be studied. It creates the obligation to conduct research only with subjects' informed consent. The principle of informed consent holds a central place in ethical justification of research involving human subjects; it was first formulated in 1947, in the Nuremberg Code.

Protection of those with diminished autonomy requires that dependent or vulnerable individuals and communities be protected against being exploited or involved in studies when persons capable of making autonomous decisions would be equally suitable according to the scientific criteria of the research project.

The duty of protection is strengthened by the ethical requirements that consent, when pertinent to a study, be given freely, and that those making decisions for others have no conflict of interest and, above all, assure the protection against injury or insult (that is, nonphysical harm) of those affected by their decisions. Subject to these requirements, the protective duty may be discharged through proxy consent, or given by a responsible relative or guardian of a dependent person.

Beneficence is a general principle that includes the historical precept "do no harm," which some prefer to regard as a separate ethical principle--that of non-maleficence--and the complementary rule that an investigator should strive to maximize possible benefit and minimize possible harm. This rule, which holds a central place in the tradition of medical ethics, proscribes the intentional injury of patients and research subjects. Harm to a person or group should never be deliberately proposed, but the risk of inadvertent harm is often inescapable. Harm is not limited to the infliction of physical injury and pain, but includes, for instance, breach of confidentiality, loss of public reputation or self-esteem, and loss of faith in others, such as might arise from questions that give rise to uneasiness and suspicion. An investigator must be able to demonstrate a favorable risk-to-benefit ratio in order to conduct research, meaning that risks are reasonable in view of realistically anticipated benefits of the proposed research. The principle of beneficence is the basis of the requirement that research have a sound design and that those who conduct it must be competent both to execute the study and to assure the well-being of the subjects.

Justice is a general principle requiring that cases considered to be alike be treated alike, and that cases considered to be different be treated in ways that acknowledge the difference. The principle of justice includes the rule of *distributive justice*, which requires a fair and equitable sharing of both burdens and benefits. The research should be designed to develop knowledge that will be of benefit to the class of persons of which the subjects are representative, so that the class of persons that share the burden should receive an appropriate benefit, and the class primarily intended to benefit shares a fair proportion of the risks and burdens.

The principle of justice reinforces the principle of *respect for persons*; namely, that competent persons be adequately informed in order to make their own choices on participation in studies, but that those with impaired or diminished competence be protected against exploitation as study subjects. The principle of distributive justice is applicable within and among communities. Weaker members of communities should not bear disproportionate burdens of studies from which all members of the community are intended to benefit, and more dependent communities should not bear disproportionate burdens of studies from which all communities within a society or country are intended to benefit.

General ethical principles are applicable to both individuals and communities. *Traditional* ethics has operated between and among individuals, being concerned with individual conscience--the ways in which one person should relate to another, and the moral entitlements of each member of a community.

Ethics that concerns person-to-person interaction is called *micro-ethics*. Ethics applies also to how one community should relate to another, and how a community should treat their members (including the next generation) and members of other groups, as well as their cultural values.

Ethics that concerns group, or communal or social, actions is called *macro-ethics*. Macro-ethics is applicable particularly to epidemiological research. In certain circumstances macro-ethical responsibilities may be judged to transcend the micro-ethical.

Both micro-ethics and macro-ethics are applicable to the ethical assessment of proposed studies. Procedures that are inconsistent with micro-ethics cannot be justified simply because they are macro-ethically acceptable, and vice versa. For instance, seeking the individual consent of competent subjects to bear the significant burdens and risks of a study cannot be omitted simply on the ground that the study would benefit the community. Equally, a study that would protect autonomy is not justifiable if the class of intended subjects would not benefit from it but a class of equally suitable persons who would benefit decline, or are not invited, to serve as subjects.

Early codes of medical ethics contained no direct reference to medical experimentation. It seems that the first reference to research involving human subjects was in 1830, in an English law on experimental treatment by doctors of their patients, which required the physician to obtain the consent of the research subjects when conducting such experiments, or else the physician would be obliged to provide compensation for any injury that might arise from his adopting a new treatment. In France, Claude Bernard in 1865 postulated that a principle of medical and surgical morality was never to perform on human subjects an experiment whose outcome could only be harmful in some degree, even though the result could be very interesting scientifically and, therefore, in the interest of the health of others.

The first reference to the principles that should govern experiments on human subjects appears to be a directive issued on 29 December 1900 by the Prussian Minister of Religious, Educational, and Medical Affairs. It directed that such experiments should not be performed on minors, or persons incompetent for other reasons, or on other persons unless they had given their unequivocal consent in the knowledge of any possible harmful consequences. Moreover, only heads of clinics or other medical institutions should perform such experiments.

The most significant (and the first national) legal instrument before the Nuremberg Code was undoubtedly the Circular of 28 February 1931, of the (German) Reich Minister of the Interior. The "Guidelines for innovative therapy and scientific experiments on man," established by this circular, resulted from a controversy between the German press and the medical profession on the ethics of human experimentation. The guidelines assert that the planning and execution of new treatment had to be compatible with medical ethics and the rules of the art and science of medicine. Risk should be carefully weighed against expected benefits, and the treatment should previously have been tested by animal experiments. New treatment should not be undertaken without patients' consent. In all institutions for the care of the sick, new forms of treatment should be carried out only by the chief physician, or with his express authorization and under his full responsibility. No experiment that could be done equally as well on animals should be done on man. Experiments on the dying were contrary to medical ethics.

Obviously, those guidelines drafted in Germany sixty years ago came very close to today's ethical requirements for research involving human subjects, especially with regard to the importance of informed consent of the subject and the need for previous animal tests. It is interesting that there appears to have been no corresponding concern, or governmental action, in any other country. It is perhaps also worthy of note that in 1876 Parliament in London already had passed the Cruelty to Animals Act.

THE NUREMBERG CODE

The Nuremberg Code was the first international declaration on research involving human subjects; it was an incidental outcome of the trial of Nuremberg physicians for having experimented on prisoners (and detainees) during World War II. It includes ten principles, and gives particular attention to the concept of "voluntary consent" (informed consent) of the subject, which is stated to be "absolutely essential." The principles of the Nuremberg Code have been embodied in many subsequent ethical codes governing research involving human subjects. Perhaps the most important effect was that the Nuremberg code raised the consciousness of people everywhere about experimentation on humans, which brought this issue to the forefront of public debate, and resulted in the issuance of many international documents on the subject.

THE DECLARATION OF HELSINKI

The medical profession, represented internationally by the World Medical Association (WMA), founded in 1947, reacted immediately to the horrors that had been revealed at the trial of doctors in Nuremberg and adopted, in 1948, the Declaration of Geneva, which is considered as a modern restatement of the Hippocratic oath, relating to the practice of medicine rather than to experimentation.

In 1953 the WMA began to consider the need for professional guidelines for experiments on human beings--guidelines designed by physicians for physicians--that would be distinct from the Nuremberg Code, which had been drawn up by jurists for juridical use.

In 1964, at the Eighteenth World Medical Assembly, this resulted in the adoption of the Declaration of Helsinki, which was a set of rules to guide physicians engaged in clinical research, both therapeutic and nontherapeutic.

Important new provisions in the revised declaration were that experimental protocols for research involving human subjects should be submitted to a specially appointed independent committee for consideration, comment, and guidance; that such protocols should always contain a statement of the ethical considerations involved and should indicate that the principles enunciated in the declaration were complied with; and that reports on experimentation not in accordance with the principles laid down in the declaration should not be accepted for publication.

The Declaration of Helsinki, further revised in 1983 and 1989, provides the fundamental guiding principles for the conduct of biomedical research involving human subjects. It has been adopted, in modified but similar forms, in international texts and national legislation, and by many professional medical organizations throughout the world.

The Nuremberg Code and the revised Declaration of Helsinki are generally considered to constitute the basis of universality in the observance of ethical-moral standards of human experimentation. The Declaration of Helsinki goes much further than the Nuremberg Code in establishing guidelines for protecting the research subject. Nevertheless, they are merely sets of ethical principles--highly influential, no doubt, but lacking any legally binding authority. The rules they set forth have no means of enforcement. They express the hope, like other declarations and codes defining ethical aspects of research on human subjects, that the medical profession will behave ethically.

International ethical declarations, by their very nature, can only be general; they must satisfy all countries and cultures. Therefore, international codes alone do not guarantee adequate protection of human research subjects. National legislation is needed, as well as an international document with binding authority.

THE WHO/CIOMS INTERNATIONAL GUIDELINES

A significant occurrence in international medical research ethics was the issuance in 1982 of the WHO/CIOMS Proposed International Guidelines for Biomedical Research Involving Human Subjects.[1] The word "proposed" does not signify that the guidelines are only in draft form, pending further comment and revision; rather, they have been proposed to countries as guidelines worthy of consideration and adoption under national standards and mores. They suggest means of implementing ethical principles on a national level.

In 1978, CIOMS and WHO joined together to prepare guidelines to assist developing countries in evolving mechanisms that could ensure adherence to medical ethics in biomedical research. Their specific objectives were to develop guidelines for the establishment of ethical review procedures for research involving human subjects, to enable countries to define national policy on the ethics of medical and health research and adopt ethical standards to suit their specific local needs, and to establish adequate mechanisms for ethical review of research involving human subjects.

As was noted at the time, those who drew up the Nuremberg Code and the Declaration of Helsinki were from the West, and both the code and the declaration reflected Western ethical principles, not necessarily applicable to other cultures. Neither, as we have learned, do they take adequate account of the realities of socio-economic and political life in most of the third world.

The guidelines were endorsed in 1981 by the Executive Committee of CIOMS and the WHO Advisory Committee on Medical Research, and therefore became known as the WHO/CIOMS Guidelines. The guidelines do not have, nor are they intended to have, the character, force, or specificity of a legal text. Instead, they provide an operational approach to the ethics of medical research, a framework upon which countries that have not yet formalized their regulatory requirements for the ethical review of research protocols may build.

Perhaps the most significant contribution of the guidelines is their analysis of the problems associated with informed consent. They acknowledge that "the involvement of human subjects in biomedical research must be contingent, whenever feasible, upon freely elicited informed consent and upon liberty to withhold or withdraw collaboration at any stage without fear or prejudice." Especially in developing countries, a person may not be sufficiently aware of the implications of being a subject of an experiment to give adequately informed consent. The guidelines therefore provide a basis for determining when research involving human subjects in such circumstances can still be vindicated and, if so, "by what mechanism their welfare can be protected and the ethical propriety of the research be assured."

The guidelines go to great lengths to determine when experimentation on the groups designated as "vulnerable" may be justified. They give particular attention to children, pregnant and nursing women, and the mentally ill. As regards community-based research, I quote: "all possible means should be used to inform the community concerned of the aims of the research, the advantages expected from it, and any possible hazards or inconveniences." Although the ultimate decision to undertake the research should rest with the responsible public-health authority, "if feasible, dissenting individuals should have the option of withholding their participation."

The guidelines suggest that, in developing countries, trusted community leaders should decide, on behalf of poorly informed and vulnerable prospective research subjects, whether they should become research subjects. This use of proxy consent is sometimes criticized on the grounds that there should be no discrimination between one population and another, and that the fundamental principle must remain that only a person's individual consent can properly justify involvement as a subject of biomedical research. The guidelines indicate that the intermediary should explain clearly to prospective research subjects that participation is entirely voluntary, and that they may abstain or withdraw from an experiment at any time.

Nevertheless, defects were recognized in the concept of "voluntary informed consent." It could not be regarded "as an exclusive means of protecting the human rights and welfare of research subjects." It must be complemented by prospective ethical review. By requiring prospective ethical review of all protocols of research involving human subjects, the guidelines are designed to ensure the same rights as those protected under Principle 1 of the Nuremberg Code, but, at the same time, provide for exceptions to the absolute requirement of informed consent in instances where, although consent may not be obtainable, experimentation on human subjects may still be ethically and morally justified.

The guidelines depart from previous international codes in two other significant ways. They consider the problems associated with externally funded research. They point out that such research implies two ethical imperatives: that the initiating or funding agency submit the research protocol to ethical review, ensuring that the ethical standards applied should be no less exacting than they would be for research carried out in the country of the agency; and that, after the agency has obtained ethical approval, the appropriate authorities of the host country should, by means of an ethical review committee or otherwise, satisfy themselves that the proposed research meets their own ethical requirements.

The guidelines pay special attention to externally funded research. This is due, in part, to the risk that investigators might subserve the interests of an external (foreign) funding agency or country rather than those of the host country. Also, foreign investigators and sponsors might not understand adequately local mores, customs, and legal systems. Lack of long-term commitment to research subjects and withdrawal of research workers on completion of their task often result in local disillusionment, and lack of accountability often precludes any form of compensation for injury due to research. Most disturbing, it was recognized that standards applied when foreign agencies carried out research in developing countries were often less stringent than those that would be applied had the research been performed in their own countries.

The guidelines are also the first international code to consider the subject of compensation of research subjects for injury sustained as a result of participation. They state that any volunteer subjects involved in medical research who may suffer injury as a result of their participation are entitled to financial or other assistance so as to compensate them fully for any temporary or permanent disability. Subjects of experiments need merely to establish a causal relationship between the investigation and the injury; they do not have to show negligence or lack of a reasonable degree of skill on the part of the investigator.

UPDATING THE WHO/CIOMS GUIDELINES

Since the publication in 1982 of the proposed guidelines, progress in science and biomedical technology has created an urgent need to update the recommendations; accordingly, CIOMS, again with the cooperation of WHO, has recently undertaken their revision.[2] Also required are similar guidelines applicable to the ethics of epidemiological research; and CIOMS, together with WHO, has developed international guidelines for Ethical Review of Epidemiological Studies.[3]

The need to update the proposed guidelines and to complement them with regard to epidemiological research has been highlighted by the HIV/AIDS pandemic and the imminent commencement of trials of candidate HIV vaccines and treatment drugs involving large communities in many parts of the world. New vaccines and drugs, not only for HIV infection but also for many other health problems affecting third-world countries will be developed in first-world countries. They must be tested on third-world populations, and this requirement creates a tension between the methods or procedures to be used and the ethical principles of autonomy, beneficence, and justice, and respect for human dignity. This is why the proposed guidelines must be updated and also why there is a need for international ethical guidelines for epidemiology.

There are also other considerations--sociocultural as well as ethical--that have to do with the socioeconomic and political realities of the third world. In the typical third-world country the poor, who represent the vast majority of the population, are helpless. They tend to submit to the will or decision of anybody who appears more powerful than themselves. They regard researchers as more powerful because they appear more knowledgeable. There is also the problem of the unjust nature of many third-world countries. Accountability is rare. Corruption is common. Even people who are better off and well educated may have no mechanisms of redress through the judicial system.

There are vast inequities in the form and distribution of health services, and in access to the health services. Often, serious health needs are not met.

In the circumstances of unjust societies, which constitute much of the third world, it is justice that is most at issue. Justice calls for universal access to health services, that is, equity in the development of health services as a principal objective of national development, and for care according to need.

To apply the ethical principle of justice, the health authority must define who will be reached with services, what are their problems and needs, what are the causes or determinants of their diseases, and what services will they need; provision must be made for communities to express their views; the services need to be monitored and evaluated, and extended or modified. Epidemiology, including epidemiological research, is essential to these tasks. Thus epidemiology is a prerequisite for ethical action in the health field; and at the same time, it must be applied, both as a research tool and as a form of public-health practice, in accordance with ethical principles. For epidemiological, community-based research in underdeveloped communities, informed consent is, in general, not practicable. Proxy consent when it is relied upon is a form of permission, rather than informed consent. In these circumstances, the responsibility to observe justice and beneficence is all the more that of the investigator and the investigating or research agency.

Ideally, the investigator or investigating group would protect the community from being used as merely a communal research specimen. This would imply (1) a degree of trust between the researchers and the subjects, and (2) the notion of moral autonomy of researchers (in a context where human relations must be viewed in the context of social hierarchies and class differences).

Small islands of the first world exist in third-world countries, just as deprived communities can be found in the first world. Each developing country has its own North. Research workers, whether biomedical or epidemiological, generally belong to these first-world islands, and their attitudes toward their third-world compatriots will affect the application of the ethical principle of autonomy, or respect for self- determination. Also, third-world researchers are often trained in the first world, and maintain their identity with, and the values of, this region; resulting in cultural and social alienation from their own communities. Yet, as researchers, they can claim to speak on behalf of all, while in reality rendering the majority voiceless.

The research subjects themselves could be the protectors of the community. This would imply equality, and mutual respect and confidence, between subjects and researchers. Could the protectors be the parents or other family members or guardians or friends of research subjects? They are also members of the deprived communities.

In such conditions, the role of the ethical review committee is crucial. It must be able to function objectively, even courageously at times, if a principal investigator is a powerful person who tends to pay scant attention to ethical principles and to expect rubber-stamp approval of a research protocol. The review committee must be sure that epidemiological studies are not another means of reinforcing the chronic deprivation and the helplessness engendered by the socioeconomic and cultural realities, and the distribution of power that is characteristic of many communities. They must not be another expression of the hierarchical power structure, and of the ad hoc nature of decision making that is characteristic of many communities. Epidemiologists can obtain useful data, but may find it too difficult in the circumstances to apply the principle of benefi-cence, and there may be no one to object.

Consider, for instance, the use of third-world communities for genetic research and the mapping of the human genome. Third-world communities, because of their large families, are considered essential for the construction of pedigrees of families with genetic defects. It is easy to see, and to say, that this research will have a beneficial impact on humanity as a whole. We can see that for a number of genetic diseases it will prove, in the short and medium terms, to be of benefit to affected families in the first world, who are served by health-care systems that function more or less as they were designed to function. But in much of the third world, especially in the least developed countries, health systems exist on paper only: they are, rather "nonsystems." There are no ways of ensuring that communities used as research subjects obtain any beneficence as a consequence. In the long term, perhaps, the descendants of the families who are used for genetic research today will benefit.

Another area with ethical overtones is the transfer, from industrialized to developing countries, of health-research technology, as well as the products of industrialized-country health-related research. The values attached to medical research in developed countries are professional values, related largely to the care of individual patients. However, in the transfer to developing countries of research and health-care technologies, researchers and physicians are relating to groups or to whole populations. The questions then arise: What does the concept of beneficence mean in these circumstances? Whose autonomy is controlling, and who determines it? Especially when commercial interests (or even national interests) are involved, we have to ask which value's system is operating--that of the market-place or that of professional ethics? Beneficence can become medical paternalism or commercial advantage, which are in conflict with the ethical principle of autonomy. Decisions may be made without respect for human dignity.

Technologies are not value-free. When technologies are transferred, values also get transferred. A technology may take on new, and perhaps unanticipated and even unwanted characteristics in the population and culture to which it is transferred. It may carry with it values that the receiving population does not want but cannot avoid. For example, in-vitro fertilization is associated with particular attitudes toward health, such as that infertility is a disease, not a misfortune or a moral judgement. Yet, according to some religious beliefs, infertility may be viewed as God's will, perhaps as a punishment for premarital sexual promiscuity.

CONCLUSION

Clearly, the third-world circumstances in which the guidelines are intended to be applied are often intimidating. There is no doubt that these guidelines will not be, or cannot be, observed to the letter and in all conditions. We can only strive continuously, by the active involvement of scientists, health professionals, philosophers, lawyers, and theologians in international, intercultural, and interdisciplinary dialogue, to ensure that the spirit of the guidelines will gradually come to permeate all of biomedical and epidemiological research, for the benefit of all of humanity. This is in line with the International Dialogue on Health Policy, Ethics, and Human Values, which is a continuing program of

CIOMS, designed to strengthen national capacities for addressing and making decisions about the ethical and human-values issues involved in health policy, and to pursue deeper understanding of human values across cultural and political lines.

NOTES

1   *Proposed International Guidelines for Biomedical Research Involving Human Subjects* (Geneva, Switzerland: CIOMS, 1982).
2   *International Ethical Guidelines for Biomedical Research Involving Human Subjects* (Geneva, Switzerland: CIOMS, in press).
3   *International Guidelines for Ethical Review of Epidemiological Studies* (Geneva, Switzerland: CIOMS, 1991).

Part IV

Use of Embryos and Fetuses

19

The Status and Uses of Early Human Developmental Stages

Clifford Grobstein

The focus of this chapter is on the moral and legal status of early human developmental stages, with emphasis on how these stages should be treated in laboratories and in clinical practice. This chapter, along with the others in this book, illustrate how diverse topics in ethics have become. With regard to the topic of research on early human development, this chapter will direct attention to the moral considerations that exert external directive pressure on research, its funding, and its outcomes.

To demonstrate the effect of external pressure on human developmental research, one need only examine a computer printout of the titles of scientific papers published in the last decade by authors in the United States. The very limited number of entries dealing with humans--as compared with other species such as mouse, chick, frog, or sea urchin--is immediately obvious.

Possible reasons for the small number of papers based on humans are also obvious; for example, the limited opportunities to detect developmental stages within the human uterus. What is not so immediately obvious is the extremely limited funding (approaching zero) currently available from US federal sources for studies on early human developmental stages. Moreover, the dearth of such funds clearly is not accidental; rather it is traceable to deliberate policy of the Federal Department of Health and Human Services (HHS). This policy has been in operation through the 1980s and, only now, at the beginning of the 1990s, is it beginning to be seriously challenged. In effect, as we enter the last decade before a new millennium, the existing funding pattern strongly suggests that understanding of early human development is of far less interest and importance than that of other species such as, say, the mouse.

Moreover, reference to the next millennium is not incidental. I refer to it because in this research area religious teachings exert significant pressure on US funding--even though the issues involved are certainly not solely religious, and teachings of various religions are hardly always concordant on the matters involved. In fact, the varied views on abortion, whether or not these stem from religion, are more directly influential in exerting pressure on funding. Defenders of current restrictive policies on funding for research on early human developmental stages argue that because human abortuses constitute a possible source of study materials, increases in the number of authorized and funded early human studies will promote a higher frequency of abortion. To others, aware of the issue, this argument is tenuous at best; it is little more persuasive than the suggestion that wider research use of adult human tissues will increase the frequency of capital punishment. In both instances, an unjustified conflation of unsubstantiated assertions is claimed to demonstrate causal connections that are then advanced as though they were objective fact.

Rather than such loose logic, what seems to be needed at this point is careful evaluation of the potential gains and losses if early human developmental stages were more accessible to scientific study. I will provide an appraisal along these lines, based on a preliminary analysis which, persuasive to me, proves that under appropriate oversight and with suitable safeguards early human developmental stages should be available to gain otherwise unobtainable important new knowledge.

To assist in making this case, let me first provide as brief essential background several major relevant landmarks in prenatal human development. A critical feature, traceable to our mammalian heritage, is of course internal gestation or pregnancy, a phenomenon of enormous consequence for humanity as a whole but having special impact on women.

The human reproductive process normally begins with insemination of a woman by a man culminating in fusion of two cells (egg and sperm), one from each parent, to produce a single zygote cell. This process of making one from two (*fusion* o. technically *syngamy*) seems to move in the wrong direction for reproduction, but is an essential preliminary step for two reasons: it activates the developmentally quiescent egg to initiate development; and it provides to the zygote a new and unique genetic constitution based on contributions from both parents. The new joint genome derives from pairing of chromosomal half-sets contributed by each of the parents, and it establishes the zygote as a new generation; that is, the zygote is genetically a new formulation capable of producing a lineage of like cells in a multicellular individual.

However, the significance of these facts as stated are the subject of major controversy and, from my point of view, are substantially misinterpreted by some commentators who insist on regarding the resulting genetic individual as immediately equivalent to the total individuality of an adult. Accordingly, these commentators declare the zygote to be a "person" in the full moral and legal sense. Other commentators, however, reject this notion as naive and misguided, pointing out that--like the preformationism of more than a century ago--the interpretation grossly miniaturizes and distorts the significance of the subsequent developmental process.

The fact, of course, is that during development the established genetic individuality is translated and transformed through step-wise expression into the much more complex reality of the new generation. The zygote does have important characteristics beyond those of either egg or sperm alone. But the zygote also lacks many key features of a person, which are readily identified in a newborn and even more clearly in an adult.

To be more specific (and extrapolating from studies on other species) the single-celled zygote is not yet even committed to becoming one individual. As it divides to form a small cluster of cells, each derived cell--if separated from the others--can make a whole new individual. The result is equivalent to natural twinning, which, of course, occurs with low but regular frequency in human development and produces litters of genetically identical individuals in armadillos. Genetic individuality, therefore, is not the same as developmental individuality; instead, the one precedes the other.

Furthermore, as cell division proceeds, the many cells produced aggregate as a collective that develops a central fluid-filled cavity within an outer cellular peripheral wall. By this stage, the developing entity has normally travelled down the oviduct and arrived in the uterus. There, its outer cells interact with the uterine lining, leading to its implantation or incorporation into the uterine wall. In this process, the peripheral cells of the developing entity do not become part of, or contribute to, the embryo proper--defined as the direct precursor to the new individual-to-be. Rather, the outer cells of this stage contribute to the early placenta--the organ of exchange with the mother--which normally is discarded at birth.

Therefore, the cellular aggregate produced by early divisions of the zygote is better referred to as a pre-embryo than as an embryo. It is only somewhat later that the actual precursor cells of the embryo--and the eventual human adult-- become conspicuously separate from the so-called trophoblast (feeding layer), which contributes to the placenta. (Interestingly, the trophoblast cells sometimes escalate on their own, undergoing malignant transformation, and take the life of either the mother, the offspring, or both.)

What should be the status of the developing entity of the pre-embryonic stage? I prefer the following tentative approach to this important and difficult question. By virtue of its earlier developmental activation, the pre-embryo has potential to become a person in the full sense. This means that it has among its alternative futures possible maturation into a person. It is, in this sense, a pre-person and this must be taken into account in its treatment and status.

What might such a status entail? First, since we should and do attach very high value to persons (in part because the category includes each of us as a self) and pre-persons are the only source of persons, every feasible opportunity and priority should be provided to pre-persons to continue their development to personhood. However, this does not require and does not mean that pre-persons are automatically and immediately persons. Rather, it means that appropriate formulation of the status and rights of pre-persons is a task of high priority, taking into account the status and rights of the mother.

Second, pre-persons, as genetic individuals, are members of the kinship network of both of their parents. In the absence of the genetic parents as decisionmakers at a critical time, an agreed-upon procedure for surrogate custodianship should exist within each human community, whether it is applied to a particular subgroup (family) or to a larger community having a reliably stable consensus within it.

Third, if acceptable custodianship based on kinship has not been provided for a given pre-embryo, it should become the responsibility of a designated public authority, which may appoint a trustee to make suitable decisions on behalf of the pre-person, with priority given as indicated in the preceding first principle.

Fourth, if all possibilities for providing continued development to personhood have been exhausted, a pre-person may be made available for other purposes, approved under rules to be formulated and monitored by a publicly responsible oversight body.

Fifth, it is assumed that such pre-persons will be maintained in an optimal frozen state pending disposition--but that they will not be so maintained for periods longer than one year unless accumulating experience indicates otherwise. Careful records should be maintained for all individual pre-embryos so as to allow modification of the one-year preliminary recommendation in response to cumulative experience.

These principles are intended to apply to pre-embryos as pre-persons, the developmental stage most often dealt with in clinical centers providing in-vitro fertilization and related techniques for treating subfertile couples. This set of applications does not, however, exhaust the growing possibilities for beneficial intervention during development in utero, whether the benefit be to the mother or the offspring. There is, therefore, growing need for greater scientific understanding of both embryonic and fetal development to support these clinical possibilities.

Thus, the first point made earlier with respect to the status of pre-embryos is equally valid for embryos--it is essential both to protect their potential as pre-persons and to better understand the nature and properties of such potential. We need therefore to define the status of embryos so that their pre-personhood is appropriately respected, while allowing knowledge about them to be effectively expanded.

The embryonic period can be defined as beginning with the appearance of the head-to-tail body axis and extending to the onset of bodily movement at six to seven weeks. The main body axis is first recognized by appearance of the so-called primitive streak in the cup-shaped layer of cells which, ten to fourteen days after fertilization, represents the nascent embryo. Shortly thereafter, in line with and ahead of the primitive streak, the neural folds appear as the first visible precursor of the central nervous system and the brain.

There follows, in regular sequence in relation to the neural axis, the appearance of various organ rudiments, each an aggregate of increasing numbers of cells undergoing complex interactions and behaviors. Included, for example, are pulsations that begin near the mid-line of the embryonic axis, as the double tubular heart rudiment commences its beat and embryonic circulation is initiated. Subsequently, other organ rudiments appear in relation to the embryonic axis--rudimentary eyes, ears, limbs, spinal cord, brain, and so forth. By six to seven weeks, neuromuscular connections have been established in the neck region sufficient to support primitive turning movements of the head. This is a reasonable marker for the transition from primary organogenesis of the embryo to fetal growth and maturation, which continues on to birth and beyond.

Movement, particularly when it seems purposeful, has significant impact on observers; accordingly, at the much later time of quickening, this was a traditional clinical sign of advancing pregnancy and fetal well-being. Today, embryonic movement is visible to ultrasonography as early as six to seven weeks of gestation and affords welcome testimony about fetal welfare. Moreover, movements imply a significant level of maturation, including the presence of receptors, neural transmitters, and effectors such as muscles. Thus movement as behavior, even when rudimentary, becomes a potential form of communication and thus an indicator of internal state that may later include the beginnings of sensation, awareness, and discomfort--all assumed to require at least minimal brain function.

With these developments, concern legitimately rises about influences and treatments that may evoke pain or other significant discomfort. Very much more knowledge about these matters is needed to deal intelligently and humanely with the "rights" of quasi-persons during their course to full subjective existence.

Recapitulating, although the human developmental course is gradual and cumulative, there are several fundamental horizons that are recognizable as major transitions. These include, in addition to fertilization, embryonic axis formation and onset of behavior as indicated by bodily movement. Each signals a new level of organization and integration, which can justify assignment of added value with regard to realized function and imminent social potential. In turn, such incremental value merits rising status, especially within societies committed to the worth and continuing realization of the individual. Thus fertilization, establishment of an embryonic body axis, and the beginning of behaviorally significant movements are major landmarks to be recognized in the developmental progression from zygote to pre-embryo, to embryo, and to fetus;

each a platform on which to build heightened status on the road to full personhood.

As noted earlier, fertilization clearly is a major landmark in conferring developmental activation and establishing the replicateable genetic instructions for a new generation. Later establishment of an embryonic axis creates a single multicellular entity as that entity is implanting into the uterine wall. There it will initiate intimate relationships, facilitating rich exchange of essential substances between offspring and mother. The relationship progresses in its intimacy and effectiveness during the fetal period of incremental magnitude, levels of differentiation, and accompanying integration. Integration sharply expands and is amplified through activities of the circulatory and nervous systems, each promoting and systematizing functions and behaviors of the organism as a whole.

Each step described is a substantial advance in the building of independent status for the new developing individual. But even at birth full independence as a person is still some years ahead. Nonetheless, in most contemporary societies full protection as a person is mandated for any newborn. Yet, the fetus, particularly in its early stages, is a far cry from a normal newborn, and no general consensus has been achieved on when in fetal life in utero a person definitely exists. There is, however, consensus that any fetus capable of survival after delivery ("viable") is a person from the time of delivery.

This is a currently defensible position, although it is subject to differences of interpretation and some resulting dissention. What seems clear is that there is no moment or single step when, or by which, a person in the full sense suddenly exists. Rather, a human being in the full sense gradually emerges through a series of steps, with no way of progressing immediately from a pre-person to a person. Nonetheless, each step makes a contribution, and we do not yet fully understand all of the steps or exactly how each contributes. Some steps can be clarified by study of other species, but no other species undergoes the full changes that are so diagnostic of humanity. Accordingly, current federal policy that minimizes support for research on human developmental stages--particularly on behavior and brain function--are seriously hampering scientific advance, to the detriment not only of science but of human welfare in the broadest sense.

There is no question, therefore, that important ethical issues are involved and that these must have careful consideration. But related issues of comparable difficulty have been faced in connection with the treatment of human subjects of research in general. A modus operandi was developed in the late 1970s and early 1980s. It is still in effect and appears to function successfully. But a special oversight committee appointed in HHS, specifically to evaluate and advise on ethical aspects of proposals for human developmental research, was allowed to lapse when appointments to it came up for renewal. Since departmental policy requires ethical evaluation of human developmental research proposals, federal financial support was thereby effectively cut off. Both Congress and professional organizations concerned with reproductive medicine are now seeking ways around this roadblock. Clearly needed is wider awareness that essentially ideological considerations are pinching off an important area of biomedical research--an area involving critical aspects of reproduction and development.

To summarize the problem in the context of this book, experience has taught us that a number of ethical issues regularly arise in the conduct of scientific research. At the primary level this book presents much about misrepresentation of data, the responsibilities of authorship, and the conflicts of interest that may arise when scientists function in centers of national policy or in corporate board rooms. These indeed are important issues and call for careful attention.

But there is another family of value issues that has plagued the interaction of science with society for centuries, perhaps as long as the two have existed. It has to do with the product of science rather than its methods or even its objectives. To attach value to scientific knowledge often means to detach value from what was previously thought to be reliable knowledge. Recall the fable of Adam and Eve, the blistering and still-heated battle over creationism and evolution, and the puzzled reactions to relativity, quarks, and black holes.

The firm belief that a complete person begins at conception and that, consequently, both contraception and abortion are moral equivalents to murder rests on supposed knowledge from which value now has to be detached. The much more difficult present reality that a person emerges gradually in complicated ways from a single cell is knowledge to which value now has to be firmly attached. Neither the substance of this relatively new knowledge nor the evidence that supports it is easily communicated throughout the body politic. Nonetheless, it must somehow become part of the scientific and technological literacy, which we are all urged to share more widely with the general community.

20

Ethical Limitations on the Use of the Human Fetus in Research

James Bopp, Jr.

This article discusses the ethical problems with human fetal tissue experimentation and transplantation employing tissue made available by the induced abortion of the fetus. The first section deals with the current moratorium declared by the Department of Health and Human Services (HHS) on federal funding of human fetal tissue experimentation and transplantation with tissue from induced abortions. I will discuss the two central pillars upon which the argument supporting the moratorium rests in the context of the 1975 report of the National Commission for the Protection of Human Subjects of Biomedical and Behavioral Research, the 1988 report of the NIH Panel on Human Fetal Tissue Transplantation Research, and normal ethical principles. This article also will consider recent federal legislative efforts to override the HHS moratorium. As will be demonstrated, these legislative efforts fail to incorporate sufficient safeguards to make them ethically acceptable, even assuming that some transplantation research using tissue from induced abortions could be ethically justified.

THE MORATORIUM ON FUNDING

On 2 November 1989, Louis W. Sullivan, MD, Secretary of Health and Human Services, notified William F. Raub, PhD, the Acting Director of the National Institutes of Health, that Sullivan had "decided to continue the moratorium on Federal funding of research in which human fetal tissue from induced abortions is transplanted into human recipients."[1] By this action, the Bush administration continued the policy begun by the Reagan administration.

Dr. Sullivan explained his considerations. "First, both the Administration and the Congress have made it clear that this Department in particular should not be funding activities which encourage or promote abortion." Secretary Sullivan noted legislative and administrative mandates, such as the Hyde Amendment,[2] and regulations recently promulgated pursuant to Title X,[3] as well as prohibitions in Title X[4] and Title XX[5] of the Public Health Service Act. The public policy underlying these enactments reflects a national consensus that, while abortion may have been decriminalized by the Supreme Court in *Roe v. Wade*,[6] it is not something the American public at large wishes to promote by public funding (except in the most exigent circumstances).

As discussed below, a majority of the American people clearly oppose the overwhelming number of abortions performed in this nation. Secretary Sullivan noted in his letter to Acting Director Raub that "it is significant that 18 of the 21 members of the NIH Human Fetal Tissue Transplantation Panel agreed to begin their Report with the following statement: 'It is of moral relevance that human fetal tissue has been obtained from induced abortions.' "

He then wrote:

> I am persuaded that one must accept the likelihood that permitting the human fetal research at issue will increase the incidence of abortion across the country. I am particularly convinced by those who point out that most women arrive at the abortion decision after much soul searching and uncertainty. Providing the additional rationalization of directly advancing the cause of human therapeutics cannot help but tilt some already vulnerable women toward a decision to have an abortion.

Secretary Sullivan found unconvincing the notion that "a strict wall could be erected between the abortion decision and the decision to donate fetal tissue to research" in actual practice. He wrote, "For example, because there is often a need to utilize post-mortem tissue promptly, it may be necessary to consult pregnant women before the abortion is actually performed. This will potentially influence the decision-making process, despite safeguards recommended by the NIH Advisory Panels. In addition, should the research efforts in question prove successful, a demand for aborted fetuses could be created. Pressure would then be created to produce more fetal tissue."

Secretary Sullivan concluded:

> For all these reasons, I believe that a decision to lift the moratorium would be inconsistent with the Administration and Congressional imperatives discussed above. I, however, note that interest exists in the private sector in continuing such research. Thus, whatever biomedical knowledge that may

be obtained from such research can be obtained without Federal subsidization.

The Bush administration continues to stand fast in the belief that this research is ethically compromised. Concerns raised by Assistant Secretary of Health James O. Mason include lack of consent, complicity with past abortions, the likelihood that it will encourage future abortions, creation of a powerful economic and institutional bond and mutual interest between the abortion industry and biomedical researchers, and concern over further national political turmoil over the divisive abortion issue.[7]

Declaration of the moratorium ignited a firestorm of protest in certain quarters. This article will address some of these concerns, while demonstrating why the moratorium is ethically justified.

What is at stake?

The central issue in the debate over fetal tissue research is ethics. This is necessarily so because of what is at stake. At stake are the lives of unborn human beings and, potentially, the lives of persons who could be medically treated with fetal tissue.

In 1975, the National Commission for the Protection of Human Subjects of Biomedical and Behavioral Research observed what is at stake in the debate over fetal research:

> Throughout the deliberations of the Commission, the belief has been affirmed that the fetus as a human subject is deserving of care and respect. Although the Commission has not addressed directly the issues of the personhood and the civil status of the fetus, the members of the Commission are convinced that moral concern should extend to all who share human genetic heritage, and that the fetus, regardless of life prospects, should be treated respectfully and with dignity.[8]

The same commission also correctly focused the debate on the ethical implications of fetal research:

> The Commission has a mandate to develop the ethical principles underlying the conduct of all research involving human subjects. . . . Scientific inquiry is a distinctly human endeavor. So, too, is the protection of individual integrity. Freedom of inquiry and the social benefits derived therefrom, as well as the protection of the individual, are valued highly and are to be encouraged. For the most part, they are compatible pursuits. When occasionally they appear to be in conflict, efforts must be made through public deliberation to effect a resolution. In effecting this resolution, the integrity of the individual is preeminent. It is therefore the duty of the Commission to specify the boundaries that respect for the fetus must impose upon

freedom of scientific inquiry. The Commission has considered the principles proposed by ethicists in relation to the exigencies of scientific inquiry, the requirements and present limitations of medical practice, and legal commentary. Among the general principles for research on human subjects judged to be valid and binding are to avoid harm whenever possible, or at least to minimize harm; to provide for fair treatment by avoiding discrimination between classes or among members of the same class; and to respect the integrity of human subjects by requiring informed consent. An additional principle pertinent to the issue at hand is to respect the human character of the fetus.[9]

The commission noted a special problem with research involving human fetuses:

> The application of the general principle enumerated above to the use of the human fetus as a research subject presents problems because the fetus cannot be a willing participant in experimentation. As with children, the comatose and other subjects unable to consent, difficult questions arise regarding the balance of risk and benefit and the validity of proxy consent.[10]

A human fetus is, without doubt, a member of the human family. Scientists first discovered that human life begins at conception about 150 years ago. Science discovered in the middle of the last century--when cell biology was discovered--that the human fetus is a unique, living, individual, human being, from the moment of conception. This scientific discovery was brought to the attention of American legislators in what was called the "physicians' crusade."[11]

Professor Victor Rosenblum set forth the historical and scientific facts concisely as follows:

> Only in the second quarter of the 19th century did biological research advance to the extent of understanding the actual mechanism of human reproduction and of what truly comprised the onset of gestational development. The 19th century saw a gradual but profoundly influential revolution in the scientific understanding of the beginning of individual mammalian life. Although sperm had been discovered in 1677, the mammalian egg was not identified until 1827. The cell was first recognized as the structural unit of organisms in 1839, and the egg and sperm were recognized as cells in the next two decades. These developments were brought to the attention of the American state legislatures and public by those professionals most familiar with their unfolding import--physicians. It was the new research finds that persuaded doctors that the old "quickening" distinction embodied in the common and some statutory law was unscientific and indefensible.[12]

That the American medical community has long understood that individual human life begins at conception is confirmed by authors from early to mid-19th century.[13]

The American states responded to advances in scientific knowledge about the unborn--brought to them by the physicians' crusade with its message that individual human life begins at conception and not quickening (as formerly believed)--by enacting abortion statutes pushing the legal protection of preborn humans back to the moment of conception. Twenty-six of the thirty-six states had laws against abortion by the end of the Civil War, as did six of the nine territories.[14] These abortion laws were designed to protect unborn human beings and not just women seeking abortion.[15] Abortion was illegal in the other states and territories under the inherited English common law, and all enacted statutory protection soon after the Civil War.

Thus, the principle in American statutory law for over a century and in our inherited English common law for centuries is that the law has protected the unborn from the moment when the science of the day believed that individual human life had begun.[16]

Some advocates of fetal tissue transplantation research, however, while acknowledging that the human fetus is a member of the species homo sapien, do not believe that biological humanness is enough. They argue that, because of the early development of the human fetus, it is not deserving of the respect of a human person and, thus, the taking of its life is not entitled to the same concern as an adult.[17] This view weighs the personhood and therefore the protection of human life on a relative scale, assigning value based on the "quality of life," not simply existence, as an individual human being. By contrast, the traditional view of our society has been the "sanctity of human life" view, which asserts that each individual human life is worthy of societal protection, regardless of the value some other human may assign to the life in question. The traditional view of the sanctity of human life has been historically embraced by Judaism, Christianity, and other religions, but it is an ancient tradition apart from these religions and has independent secular justification. These sanctity-of-human-life traditions consider all human life as inherently valuable and warranting protection.[18]

It is noteworthy that the 1975 National Commission for the Protection of Human Subjects of Biomedical and Behavioral Research eschewed such a quality-of-life ethics. Rather, it employed a biological life ethics, as evidenced in the language of its report:

Throughout the deliberations of the Commission, the belief has been affirmed that the fetus as a human subject is deserving of respect and care. Although the Commission has not addressed directly the issue of the personhood and the civil status of the fetus, the members of the Commission are convinced that moral concern should extend to all who share the human genetic heritage, and that the fetus, regardless of life prospects, should be treated respectfully and with dignity.[19]

Our society has recently been influenced by this quality-of-life ethics; that is, the view that some lives are not worth living. This quality-of-life ethics has slipped into discussions of research using tissue from induced abortions. It takes the form of calling a developing human life something other than a human being, so that the human fetus is portrayed as a pre-person not worthy of respect and protection. This is in reality a quality-of-life argument (that is, unless a human organism has achieved a certain quality level, it is not a person). Those who would ask whether a human fetus has reached a certain functioning level--such as, does it have brain waves?--before recognizing it as human, are really using a quality-of-life standard. Quality-of-life valuations require artificial differentiations among human beings, based upon "quality" achieved rather than the inherent nature of the being.

One of the problems with a developmental stage, quality-of-life evaluation of who qualifies as "human," is that embryos and fetuses are not frozen in time. Those who would base value on developmental stages assume that time has stopped so that we are justified in judging the fetus at the time that the termination of its life is under consideration. Of course, the fetus is not frozen in time. It is on a journey that will lead to full adulthood--absent natural or artificial intervention. Thus, while a one-celled fertilized egg and an amoeba are similar in certain respects, they are fundamentally different. The human zygote is but passing through one stage to another, leading inexorably to a full human adult. The amoeba has already reached its full potential. Thus, one of the inherent qualities of the human fetus at every stage is its potential, a quality that makes it illegitimate to judge its value only on its current developmental stage.

Therefore, at stake in the debate over fetal tissue research are the lives of unborn human beings, which are "deserving of care and respect."[20] If fetal tissue research and transplantation therapy promote the taking of the lives of human fetuses by abortion that would not otherwise occur, then fetal tissue transplantation involves the unethical taking of human life.

THE CASE FOR THE MORATORIUM

Even assuming that induced abortion remains legal and fetal tissue transplantation proves effective, fetal tissue transplantation research with tissue from induced abortions is still ethically compromised and thus should not be pursued.

The moratorium was premised on the notion that using human fetal tissue obtained from induced abortions is unethical. The argument supporting the moratorium rests upon two central pillars. These two ethical grounds are (1) respect for the bodily integrity of another and (2) the proscription against taking the life of one person to benefit another. The following is the case in favor of the moratorium.

Pillar 1: Respect for Human Bodily Integrity

The first pillar in the case in favor of the moratorium is the ethical recognition that all human beings merit respect for their bodily integrity. The United States Supreme Court, in *Winston v. Lee*,[21] held that an individual has an interest in "personal privacy and bodily integrity" sufficiently strong to prevent a state from compelling a criminal defendant to submit to minor surgery to remove a bullet. The Court characterized such action as a "severe" invasion of his bodily integrity. Similarly, the Court has found that even medical procedures that are not physically invasive, such as urinalysis or breathalyzer tests, implicate concern for an individual's bodily integrity.[22] In the case of *Union Pacific Ry. Co. v. Botsford*,the Supreme Court declared:

> No right is more sacred, or is more carefully guarded, by the common law, than the right of every individual to the possession and control of his own person, free from all restraint or interference of others, unless by clear and unquestionable authority of law.[23]

In the medical field, the common law has protected the right of bodily integrity by making unconsented intrusions upon bodily integrity into a battery.[24] The law has also developed the doctrine of informed consent, based on this notion of an individual's right to bodily integrity.[25]

Thus, one of our pre-eminent legal principles, based on ethical concerns, protects persons from unconsented-to violations of their bodily integrity.

Termination of an unborn human life by abortion violates the principle of respecting the bodily integrity of other human beings. Clearly, no consent is obtained from the fetus about to be aborted. Clearly, dismemberment, chemical poisoning, or removal of a human fetus from the womb prior to viability violates the bodily integrity of the fetus so assaulted. Therefore, abortion constitutes a violation of this ethical principle.

The next question, of course, is whether there is some justification for this violation that falls within traditionally accepted exceptions to the principle. The bodily integrity of one person may be violated, to some degree, in order to protect other persons or in the interests of justice. Thus, invasion of a person's body has been justified (for example, in cases where there is need to prevent the spread of a plague by vaccination).[26] However, no such traditional exception is applicable to allow invasion of the bodily integrity of the fetus. Of course, where a mother's life is at risk, society has historically allowed abortion to preserve her life. However, such abortions are rare, and most are performed for reasons less grave. In fact, most abortions are done for reasons far less serious than those abortions of which the vast majority of Americans approve, as discussed below.

Thus, the vast number of abortions are performed in unjustified violation of the principle that a human fetus, as a genetically complete member of the human family, is entitled to have his or her bodily integrity respected. Abortion is, therefore, objectionable under traditional ethical standards.

Research with human fetal tissue from induced abortion is also violative of the principle of respect for the bodily integrity of another. This is so because there is no valid consent to research on the fetus and because of the problems of being in complicity with past and future abortions, legitimating the abortion industry, and diminishing respect for human life.

While people live, they have the right to consent or not consent to medical experimentation on their person, and they have the right to consent or not to the donation of their body tissue. By law, individuals may also leave enforceable directives for disposition of their property or person after their death. By these means, one may leave one's wealth to children and one's body to a medical school. However, certain restrictions apply. By law, certain formalities must be complied with before the enforcement of one's wishes is possible.

Furthermore, the intended beneficiary may be stripped of the intended beneficence by misconduct. For example, the beneficiary of a last will and testament who kills a parent to inherit the fortune under that will will receive nothing if convicted. An executor who acts contrary to the last will and testament may be replaced, just as a trustee of a testamentary trust who violates the terms of the trust may be removed. These persons have a fiduciary duty to act according to the wishes of the deceased.

Similarly, family members have a fiduciary duty to a deceased family member to provide for burial. This is not a property interest, for when a human individual dies, family members have no property right in the body of the deceased.[27] The family of the deceased, beginning in preference with the next-of-kin, does possess a "quasi-property right in a dead body . . . arising out of their duty to bury their dead, and the right to maintain an action to recover damages for any outrage, indignity, or injury to the body of the deceased."[28] However, "rights in a dead body exist ordinarily only for purposes of burial and, except with statutory authorization, for no other purpose."[29]

The Uniform Anatomical Gift Act (UAGA) broadens this "burial only" authority with regard to organ donation from deceased relatives. It is designed to facilitate organ donation and to prevent the forcible seizure of organs without consent. The UAGA requires that donation occur only after the donor has given voluntary and informed consent. If this is not possible, the donation may still be made if consent is given by a relative acting as a proxy.[30] Proponents of fetal research have attempted to "fit" the donation of fetal organs into the framework of the UAGA so that the back-up provision, consent by proxy, can save the donation from failing due to the obvious lack of consent by the fetus.[31]

However, the UAGA does not legitimate the retrieval of fetal tissue for three reasons. First, this statute is premised on the assumption that the relative acting as a proxy will genuinely care for the deceased and act in his or her best interests. Second, the UAGA assumes that the proxy will not be responsible for the death of the deceased. Third, when a proxy consents to the donation of organs from an adult cadaver, it is only after the cadaver has been declared dead. The proxy only plays a role in organ donation after death and only if the deceased person has not previously expressed his or her desires. When a woman rejects her maternal role by aborting her child, however, she forfeits any maternal fiduciary interests she possessed.[32] She is not the caring proxy that the drafters of the UAGA envisioned, but is instead the agent of death.[33]

Ethicist Albert R. Jonsen has recognized the shortcomings of the UAGA fetal-research analogy, and has admitted that the consent of the mother is suspect.[34] Yet Jonsen concludes that this lack of consent does not matter because "the genuine possibility of significant benefit to others overrides any secondary purposes that consent and permission might have."[35] Similarly, John A. Robertson, a professor at the University of Texas School of Law and a leading advocate of fetal tissue research, has suggested that research conducted on fetuses while still alive in the womb would pose no ethical dilemma for him if it were necessary to achieve further benefits.[36] This approach could easily gain support from other utilitarian thinkers who will deduce, "If one is going to die anyway, why not get some good out of it?" However, society has rejected the idea of collectively profiting from the destruction of others. As Kathleen Nolan has stated:

> Society does not generally allow those directly involved in the death of another to determine the disposition of the body. For example, while some countries tolerate capital punishment, there is widespread reluctance to transplant organs from prisoners executed by the state. (Mainland China provides an exception that serves only to prove the rule.) The reluctance to obtain organs in this fashion can be explained by noting that the decision to execute someone, no matter how well justified, is a tremendously weighty and complicated one. Such judgments are overwhelmingly difficult in the best of circumstances, so that any feature which would introduce unnecessary bias or conflict of interest should be diligently avoided.[37]

A case decided by the Illinois Supreme Court, *Curran v. Bosze*, establishes a key point relating to consent for tissue taken from a child for the benefit of another.[38] In that case, the father of twins, who were three and one-half years of age and in the custody of their mother, sought a court order requiring them to submit to bone marrow harvesting for the benefit of their half-brother who suffered from leukemia. As the twins were minors, the father sought to assert the doctrine of consent by substituted judgment, which was held inapplicable because it applied to considering the prior expressions of an individual to determine his or her wishes with regard to life-prolonging treatment. The court held "that a parent or guardian may give consent on behalf of a minor daughter or son for the child to donate bone marrow to a sibling, only when to do so would be in the minor's best interest."[39] The application to abortion is clear: it is not in the best interest of a fetus to have his or her tissue donated to another for the donee's benefit, especially where the fetus must lose his or her life for the donation to be effected. Therefore, a mother cannot give a valid consent for the donation of tissue from a fetus she carries because the donation is not in the best interest of the fetus.

Oddly enough, some argue that the fetus, as a member of the human community, has some duty to the rest of the human family to make the best possible use of its truncated life, which duty may serve as a basis for the necessary consent.[40] It is ironic that an unborn child can be aborted because it is not considered, by some, a legally protectable member of the human community, but when convenient, its obvious humanity is trotted out to public view. Of course, it is precisely because the fetal tissue is human tissue that it has possible use in transplantation; by the very act of selecting and using fetal tissue, researchers acknowledge that the fetus is a member of the human family. Kathleen Nolan aptly responds: "In the setting of elective abortion a cruel irony thus emerges: fetuses that have been excluded from membership in the human community by a societally sanctioned maternal decision to abort now have obligations to that same community because of membership in it."[41] Clearly, there is no valid consent from the fetus, just as there is no ethically valid maternal consent to the use of fetal tissue from induced abortions.

Pillar 2: No Human Being May Be Killed to Benefit Another

A second pillar of the case for the moratorium is the ethical principle that no human being may be killed to benefit another. One may not kill another to benefit oneself or a third party. This principle is expressed by criminal laws against homicide, which is killing another human being. While a strictly defined and limited exception to the homicide prohibition is made for self-defense, this exception does not cover taking the life of one human being to recover parts or tissue for the benefit of another.[42]

An English case dealt directly with killing another to benefit from his tissue long before fetal tissue transplantation became potentially feasible. The case, *Regina v. Dudley*,[43] considered the guilt of two men in a life boat for killing a seventeen-year-old boy on board in order to eat his flesh and drink his blood. They were rescued by a passing ship four days after the killing took place. Both Dudley, the man who killed the youth, and Stevens, who consented to the murder although he took no active part in it, were convicted of murder. The men had been without food for twenty days, except for two tins of turnips and a turtle, which were consumed early in their ordeal. They also were without potable water, except for some occasional rain water. The court determined that the grave threat to their life by starvation and dehydration did not constitute a "necessity" defense for the taking of the innocent life of the lad and was not considered a justification for the murder.

The jury, in the Dudley case, found (1) that at the time of the murder the murderers had been without food and water for several days; (2) that the murderers spoke of their having families and that it would be better for the boy to die than one of them on this account; (3) that the boy did not consent to his death but was unable--by reason of his weakness--to resist the fatal knife thrust; (4) that the murderers "would probably not have survived to be . . . rescued" if they had not eaten the lad; (5) "that the boy, being in a much weaker condition, was likely to have died before them;" (6) "that there was no appreciable chance of saving life except by killing some one for the others to eat;" and (7) "that assuming any necessity to kill anybody, there was no greater necessity for killing the boy than any of the other[s]."

The Dudley court decided that on the law "the deliberate killing of this unoffending and unresisting boy was clearly murder, unless the killing can be justified by . . . necessity." The court noted that there is no "absolute or unqualified necessity to preserve one's life." In fact, "it may be the plainest and highest duty to sacrifice it" under certain circumstances. The court noted the awful danger of allowing a necessity defense to the murder of an innocent person:

"Who is to be the judge of this sort of necessity? By what measure is the comparative value of lives to be measured? Is it to be strength, or intellect, or what? It is plain that the principle leaves to him who is to profit by it to determine the necessity which will justify him in deliberately taking another's life to save his own."

Noting the extremity of the temptation, the court declared: "But a man has no right to declare temptation to be an excuse, though he himself might have yielded to it, nor allow compassion for the criminal to change or weaken in any manner the legal definition of the crime."

The court proceeded to convict Dudley and his consenting accomplice of murder and to sentence them to death, a sentence reduced by the Crown to a period of imprisonment in the exercise of its prerogative of mercy. Thus, even though the tissue of this English boy was desperately needed by his shipmates to save their lives, the court declared their act morally and legally reprehensible.

The principle that we don't kill others for the benefit of ourselves or another has been with the human race for as long as homicide has been forbidden by society, for in nearly every homicide, the killing is done for some benefit to someone. The universal consensus of civilized people has been that any killing of another--or anything which would aid or promote such killing--for the benefit of another is morally wrong and must be legally forbidden. Thus, we have laws against aiding and abetting the commission of a homicide, against conspiring to commit a homicide, and against soliciting someone to commit a homicide.

Successful fetal tissue transplant now is likely to cause some abortions to occur that would not have otherwise been performed because of the influence the transplantation would have on a woman considering an abortion. Thus, some unborn lives would be taken and used for transplantation who would otherwise have been carried to term. Transplantation therapy, therefore, violates the ethical principle that one may not sacrifice the life of one to benefit another. Transplantation research that would lead to this result is likewise unethical.

WHY PUBLIC FUNDS SHOULD NOT BE USED FOR RESEARCH

The moratorium on federal funding of fetal tissue transplantation research raises an additional matter beyond the ethical acceptability of such research. When government funds are involved, it becomes a matter of public policy. With regard to transplantation research, there is an established federal policy prohibiting the promotion of abortion. This is evident in the Hyde Amendment,[44] the Title X abortion regulations,[45] as well as statutory prohibitions in Title X[46] and Title XX[47] of the Public Health Service Act.

The reason Congress has refused to fund abortions is that abortion is not viewed by the American people as an inherent good. It is, at best, something that some people believe should be tolerated as a liberty. But few people would declare it a good in itself. It is at most a "necessary evil"--one not to be encouraged or promoted--while many feel that it should be substantially limited.

This is the view of the American people, as evidenced by the latest polls. The Gallup organization recently conducted a survey of public opinion regarding "Abortion and Moral Beliefs."[48] One key finding of this study reveals that 77 percent of those surveyed believe that abortion is an evil, and consider it an act of murder or the taking of human life. The study further indicated that a majority of Americans disapprove of a majority of abortions performed in this country. Of those surveyed, 25 percent disapprove of all abortions performed for any reason. An additional 49 percent oppose abortions conducted for any reasons other than (1) the protection of the life or health of the mother, (2) the termination of a pregnancy conceived in rape or incest, or (3) in the case of a serious fetal deformity. The Alan Guttmacher Institute, however, reported that most abortions are not performed for the above three reasons. Thus, the Gallup survey summarized its findings as follows, "Those who would support a woman's right to have an abortion at any time, for any reason--as allowed by *Roe v. Wade* and defended by pro-choice groups--are in the minority."

Similarly, the Supreme Court did not decide *Roe v. Wade* on the basis that abortion is an inherent good which ought to be promoted.[49] Rather, it viewed the matter as a constitutional right, arguing that regardless of its morality--the debate over which the Court noted and which debate the Court assiduously avoided--women ought to be allowed to make this decision themselves. However, in the cases regarding public funding of abortion, *Maher v. Roe*[50] and *Harris v. McRae,*[51] the Court noted that as a matter of public policy a state or the federal government could seek to promote childbirth over abortion, recognizing that opposition to abortion was based on a traditional view that abortion was morally wrong. In practice, many states and the federal government have decided to promote childbirth over abortion by not publicly funding abortion for indigent women, except in the gravest circumstances, although they fund expenses relating to childbirth. Thus, even under *Roe v. Wade*, the federal government policy of refusing to promote abortion is justified and refusal to fund fetal tissue transplantation research is an integral part of it.[52]

CAN "SAFEGUARDS" AVOID THE ETHICAL PROBLEMS?

The NIH panel made certain procedural recommendations that it believed would eliminate any possible ethical concerns because "the [possible or alleged] immorality of its source could be ethically isolated from the morality of its use in research."[53] However, the panel simply assumed--presumably under the tutelage of its panel members (such as Dr. Hoffer, a professor of pharmacology from the University of Colorado, who was one of the members of the NIH panel who endorsed federal funding of fetal tissue transplantation experimentation with human fetal tissue from induced abortions, and who is engaged in human fetal tissue transplantation research)--that the research would occur in certain ways. However, in real life, the practice is much different, as Dr. Hoffer documented in an article on the subject.[54] Because the NIH panel either ignored these real-life ethical problems or was naively unaware of them, the procedural recommendations of the report do not begin to resolve the ethical issues.

NIH PANEL REPORT PRESUPPOSITIONS

The overriding presupposition of the NIH panel was that "it was acceptable public policy to support transplant research with fetal tissue either because the source of the tissue posed no moral problem or because the immorality of its source could be ethically isolated from the morality of its use in research."[55]

The NIH panel also made the following presuppositions: (1) that the ethical character or federally funded fetal tissue experimentation could be considered apart from what was (and what would be) going on in the real world of human fetal tissue transplantation; (2) that the researcher and the recipient could be prevented from having any role (direct or through an intermediary) in inducing or performing abortions; (3) that a woman's abortion decision could be insulated from inducements (by a researcher, recipient, or intermediary) to abort to provide tissue for transplant research and therapy; (4) that the timing and method of abortion would not be influenced (by a researcher, recipient, or intermediary) by the potential uses of fetal tissue for transplantation or medical research; (5) that the fetus is always already dead tissue when tissue collectors harvest the human fetal tissues, and that researchers are only interested in fetuses after they are already dead and aborted; and (6) that it could resolve a moral issue, as it had been asked to do, by appeals to legality and potential benefit from the transplantation.

NIH PANEL REPORT "SAFEGUARDS"

On the basis of its presuppositions, the NIH panel proposed the following procedural requirements as a means of allaying the concerns of those concerned about ethical problems with federal funding of fetal tissue transplantation research:

1. The decision to terminate a pregnancy and the procedures of abortion should be kept independent from the retrieval and use of fetal tissue.
2. Payments and other forms of remuneration and compensation associated with the procurement of fetal tissue should be prohibited, except payment for reasonable expenses occasioned by the actual retrieval, storage, preparation, and transportation of the tissues.
3. Potential recipients of such tissues, as well as research and health-care participants, should be properly informed as to the source of the tissues in question.
4. Procedures must be adopted that accord human fetal tissue the same respect afforded other cadaveric human tissues entitled to respect.[56]

WHY THE SAFEGUARDS ARE NOT SAFE

In the real world of fetal tissue transplantation, researchers do not always wait until the human fetus is dead.[57] A 1987 article in the *Hastings Center Report* by a bioethicist and two researchers admitted that "the fetal brain may not yet be dead" when they extract it.[58] However, they asserted that it is "morally defensible" to harvest tissues from yet-living but "nonviable" fetuses, "if dead fetuses are not available or are not conducive to successful transplants." Fetal pain, they argued, "may be satisfactorily addressed on a practical level by using anesthesia."

A report issued by the University of Minnesota Center for Bioethics stated that in Sweden, "doctors say they have obtained brain tissue with a forceps before the fetus was suctioned out of the mother. That raises the question of whether the fetus was killed by the harvesting of brain tissue or abortion."[59] These and other aspects of the real world must be kept in mind in evaluating the presuppositions of the NIH panel.

The first error of the NIH panel was that it gave no consideration to what the research it proposed to fund would lead to in terms of actual transplantation therapy. If it is obvious, as it is from the literature, that those engaging in fetal tissue transplantation therapy are going to employ techniques (such as the live-fetus brain removal as described by Dr. Barry Hoffer)[60] that the panel apparently opposes, promoting such therapy by funding research leading to it is unethical. A second error is the NIH panel's presumption "that neither the researcher nor the recipient would have any role in inducing or performing the abortion."[61] As shown in the examples of Freed[62] and Hoffer,[63] however, researchers have definite opinions on the sort of tissue they want and how to obtain the sort of tissue they desire. In advertising for tissue, they seek tissue collected by certain techniques. Although current federal regulations prohibit researchers involved in a federally funded project from using such methods, there is no certainty that such regulations will remain in effect given enormous pressures to provide fresh tissue for recipients. Moreover, should fetal tissue transplantation research prove successful, the therapy will be conducted without federal funds, and thus the current federal regulations would not apply, leaving the therapists free to use the methods most likely to retrieve usable tissue.

Moreover, as mentioned above, there is every likelihood that abortions will be increased with the widespread knowledge of fetal tissue transplantation that already exists and will expand in the future. However, the NIH panel was not predisposed to take this threat seriously because of the belief of a majority of its members that it really did not matter whether abortions increased. In a concurring opinion to the NIH panel report written by John Robertson, a majority of the panel declared:

> If there were a substantial increase in the number of abortions, it still would not follow that fetal tissue transplant research and therapy should not occur. Given the rudimentary development of early fetuses, the potentially great benefit to recipients, and the legality of abortion, such transplants might still be ethically and legally acceptable.[64]

Robertson and nine other panel members even expressed a willingness to consider (and likely condone) maternal "donor designation of recipients and aborting for transplant purposes" if necessary to assure adequate supplies of fetal parts. This indicates that for these members (and perhaps others unwilling to sign their names to the proposition) the NIH panel recommended-procedural rules barring designated donors were not really something they believed in (Robertson states as much).[65] They were mere window dressing to obtain federal funding.

A third error of the NIH panel was its presupposition "that a woman's abortion decision would be insulated from inducements to abort to provide tissue for transplant research and therapy."[66] If fetal tissue transplantation proved successful, it would be common knowledge that fetal tissue from elective abortions would be used to save lives. This fact would influence some women to choose abortion, when otherwise they might have continued their pregnancies. Furthermore, the NIH panel would allow a woman who asks about transplantation prior to making her abortion decision to be given information on the option.[67] Thus, the notion that women will not know of the transplantation option is not credible.

The NIH panel concedes as much, although it fails to act on the logical consequences from its concession: the panel said, "It would be unrealistic not to consider the possibility that transplantation and research with fetal tissue may enter the balance of considerations of a pregnant woman in deciding whether to have an abortion . . . because transplantation and research with fetal tissue will become general knowledge; it will not be possible to keep the populace from knowing about it." The response of the NIH panel was to find that there is no inducement inherent in obtaining informed consent from a woman for use of her aborted human fetal tissue (by the giving of information which may induce her to choose abortion). However, simply defining knowledge as no inducement does not provide the sort of insulation between abortion and fetal tissue experimentation the NIH panel claims is possible.

A fourth error of the NIH panel is the presupposition that "the timing and method of abortion should not be influenced by the potential uses of fetal tissue for transplantation or medical research."[68] In real practice, the method, at least, has already been altered. If researchers could not do this under current federal regulations, there is nothing to prevent intermediaries from collecting fetal tissue in the manner that researchers, by their own admission, prefer and employ when unencumbered by the need to get federal funds.

A fifth error of the NIH panel is the presupposition that at the time when experimentation or transplantation is considered the human fetus is already dead.[69] This is not always the case; in fact, tissue collectors have been the agents of fetal death.

A sixth error of the NIH panel was its presupposition that mere appeals to the moribund legality of abortion and potential benefit to recipients could resolve the ethical issues involved in human fetal tissue transplantation research. These arguments are inadequate to warrant approval for federal funding of human fetal tissue transplantation research from induced abortions, and standard ethical principles require a contrary result. The NIH panel never really addressed the morality of the issue, but sidestepped the key issue it was to address.

In sum, rather than the ethically well-ordered world that the NIH panel presumed, the real world of human fetal tissue transplantation research is one where human fetuses are at times separated of body parts while yet living, women are willing to risk their health by using less-safe abortion procedures for the sake of suitable tissue donation, and researchers are willing to exploit unborn human beings, women, and patients with less-than-proven (and often dangerous) therapies.

Because of the flawed basis of the NIH panel report, the safeguards it proposed do not reach the real-world ethical problems of human fetal tissue transplantation research and therapy. As a consequence, the two bills building upon the NIH report do not provide any real safety to human fetuses, women seeking abortion, or human fetal tissue recipients. Even the minor safeguard of having a woman state that her abortion is not being done for purposes of fetal tissue donation--which in no way infringes on her ability to choose abortion, is done in connection with an entirely voluntary program, and does not require her to state for what reason she is having the abortion--has been rejected in the latest bill to be introduced.

Nowhere in any of the procedural recommendations is there any protection against human fetal tissue collectors actually serving as the agents of death in the real world of transplantation therapy, which may follow the federally funded research. Nowhere are third-party collectors prohibited from collection techniques, even where the tissue will be used in federally funded programs. Nowhere is there any regulation of nonfederally funded human fetal transplantation research or therapy to prevent fetal tissue collection from yet-living fetuses or to prevent using more dangerous abortion procedures to collect fresher tissue.

Nor are researchers pushing for such safeguards. Rather, researchers such as Dr. Hoffer are out collecting tissue in ways repugnant to ethics and the American public. They only offer up such limited safeguards as a way of obtaining federal funds. They don't really believe in the ethical necessity of the safeguards, and once federally funded experimentation perfects the therapy techniques, they will operate therapy programs in the way they please. By the actions of Dr. Hoffer and his colleagues, it is evident that they will practice their therapy just as they have practiced it to date--with few if any efforts to isolate abortion from research and therapy.

CONCLUSION

In sum, the risk of promoting abortion by using fetal tissue from induced abortions for transplants is too great to make it ethically acceptable. Moreover, intertwining research facilities with abortion facilities would legitimate the abortion industry and create entanglements that would further promote abortion. The complicity with the wrong done the innocent unborn humans taints the morality of using their parts, especially since there is no acceptable consent. Thus, fetal tissue transplantation research and therapy cannot be conducted ethically, and, thus, the federal government policy of not funding it is justified. Nothing in recent legislation designed to overturn the HHS moratorium alters this situation.

NOTES

1 L.W. Sullivan, letter to William F. Raub, 2 November 1989.
2 The Hyde Amendment, Pub. L. No. 100-2-2, 101 Stat. 1329-99 (1987).
3 Title X Regulations, 42 *CFR* 59.7-59.10.
4 Title X, 42 USCA 3000-6 (West 1982).

5   Title XX, 42 USCA 3002-10 (West 1982).

6   *Roe v. Wade*, 410 US 113 (1973).

7   J.O. Mason, "Should the Fetal Tissue Research Ban Be Lifted?" *Journal of National Institutes of Health Research* 2 (1990):17.

8   The National Commission for the Protection of Human Subjects of Biomedical and Behavioral Research, *Report and Recommendations: Research on the Fetus* (Washington, DC: US Dept. of Health, Education and Welfare, 1975), DHEW publication no. (OS)76-127), 61-62.

9   *Ibid.*, 63.

10   *Ibid.*, 64.

11   J.C. Mohr, *Abortion in America: The Origins and Evolution of National Policy, 1800-1900* (New York: Oxford, 1978), 147-70.

12   Senate Committee on the Judiciary, *The Human Life Bill: Hearings on S. 158 Before the Subcommittee on Separation of Powers*, 97th Cong., 1st Sess., 1981, 474 (statement of Victor Rosenblum, professor of law and political science, Northwestern University).

13   T. Cooper, *Tracts on Medical Jurisprudence* (Philadelphia: James Webster, 1819), 40; A. Dean, *Principles of Medical Jurisprudence* (Albany: Gould, Banks, 1850), 37-41; T.R. Beck, *Elements of Medical Jurisprudence*, 12th ed. (Philadelphia: J.B. Lippincott, 1863), 1:462-64.

14   J.W. Dellapenna, "The History of Abortion: Technology, Morality, and Law," *University of Pittsburgh Law Review* 40 (1979):429.

15   J.D. Gorby, "The 'Right' to an Abortion, The Scope of Fourteenth Amendment 'Personhood,' and the Supreme Court's Birth Requirement," *Southern Illinois University Law Journal* 1 (1979):16-17.

16   J.W. Dellapenna, "The Historical Case Against Abortion," *Continuity* (Spring 1989):59; Dellapenna, "The History of Abortion," 359; J.T. Noonan, Jr., "An Almost Absolute Value in History," in *The Morality of Abortion: Legal and Historical Perspectives*, ed. J.T. Noonan, Jr. (Cambridge, MA: Harvard University Press, 1970), 1.

17   Human Fetal Tissue Transplantation Research Panel (Consultants to the Advisory Committee to the Director, National Institutes of Health), *Report of the Human Fetal Tissue Transplantation Research Panel,* vol. 1 (Washington, DC: National Institutes of Health, 1988), 35, n.21.

18   "A New Ethic for Medicine and Society," *Western Journal of Medicine* 113 (1970):67-68.

19   National Commission, *Report and Recommendations*.

20   *Ibid.*

21   *Winston v. Lee*, 470 US 753 (1985).

22   See also *Skinner v. Railway Labor Executives' Ass'n*, 109 S. Ct. 1402, 1412-13 (1989); *Schmerber v. California*, 384 US 757, 772 (1966); *Rochin v. California*, 342 US 165, 173-74 (1952).

23   *Union Pacific Ry. Co. v. Botsford*, 141 US 250, 251 (1891).

24   W.P. Keeton, D.B. Dobbs, R.E. Keeton, and D.G. Owen, *Prosser & Keeton on the Law of Torts*, 5th ed. (St. Paul: West, 1984), 190.

25   *Canterbury v. Spence*, 464 F.2d 772, 780 (DC Cir. 1972), *cert. denied*, 409 US 1064 (1972).

26   *Jacobson v. Massachusetts*, 197 US 11 (1905).

27   *Dougherty v. Mercantile Safe Deposit and Trust Co.*, 387 A.2d 244, 246 n.2 (MD App. 1978).

28   *Barela v. Frank A. Hubbell Co.*, 67 NM 319, 323, 355 P.2d 133, 136 (1960).

29   *Dougherty v. Mercantile Safe Deposit and Trust Co.*, 387 A.2d 244, 246 n.2 (MD App. 1978), quoting P.E. Jackson, *The Law of Cadavers and of Burial Places*, 2d ed. (New York: Prentice-Hall, 1950).

30   "Medical Applications of Fetal Tissue Transplantation," *Journal of the American Medical Association* 263, no. 4 (1990):568.

31   J.A. Robertson, "Rights, Symbolism, and Public Policy in Fetal Issue Transplants," *Hastings Center Report* 18, no.6 (December 1988);5-12.

32   K. Nolan, "Genug ist Genug: A Fetus Is Not a Kidney," *Hastings Center Report*, 18, no.6 (December 1988):13-19.

33   K. Nolan, "The Use of Embryo or Fetus in Transplantation: What There Is to Lose," *Transplantation Proceedings* 22 (1990):1028-29.

34   C.Q. Gelernter, "Former Jesuit Priest Is an Ethics Expert," *Seattle Times*, 7 March 1988, p. F2.

35   *Ibid.*

36   J.A. Robertson, "Fetal Tissue Transplants," *Washington University Law Quarterly* 66 (1988):443-98.

37   Nolan, "The Use of Embryo or Fetus in Transplantation."

38   *Curran v. Bosze*, 566 N.E.2d 1319 (IL 1990).

39   *Ibid.*, 1331.

40   M.B. Mahowald, J. Silver, and R.A. Ratcheson, "The Ethical Options in Transplanting Fetal Tissue," *Hastings Center Report* 17, no.1 (February 1987): 9-15.

41   Nolan, "Genug ist Genug."

42   "Homicide," *American Jurisprudence,* vol. 40, 2nd ed. (Rochester: Lawyers Co-operative Publishing Co., 1968).

43   *Regina v. Dudley*, 15 Cox C.C. 624, 14 Q.B.D. 273 (1884).

44   Pub. L. No. 100-202, 101 Stat. 1329-99 (1987).

45   42 *CFR* 59.7-59.10.

46   42 USCA 3000-6 (West 1982).

47   42 USCA 3002-10 (West 1982).

48   *The Gallup Organization, Abortion and Moral Beliefs: A Survey of American Opinion--Executive Summary* (Chicago: Americans United for Life, 1991).

49   *Roe v. Wade*, 410 US 113 (1973).

50   *Maher v. Roe*, 432 US 464 (1977).

51   *Harris v. McRae*, 448 US 297 (1980).

52 *Roe v. Wade*, 410 US 113 (1973).

53 Human Fetal Tissue Transplantation Research Panel, *Report*, 2.

54 O. Lindvall, S. Rehncrona, P. Brundin, *et al.*, "Human Fetal Dopamine Neurons Grafted into the Striatum in Two Patients with Severe Parkinson's Disease," *Archives of Neurology* 46 (1989): 615-16.

55 Human Fetal Tissue Transplantation Research Panel, *Report*, 2.

56 *Ibid.,* 1.

57 Lindvall, Rehncrona, Brundin, *et al.*, "Human Fetal Dopamine Neurons."

58 Mahowald, Silver, and Ratcheson, "The Ethical Options."

59 Quoted in Statement of Rep. Thomas J. Bliley, Jr., before the House Subcommittee on Aging, 2 April 1990.

60 Lindvall, Rehncrona, Brundin, *et al.*, "Human Fetal Dopamine Neurons."

61 Human Fetal Tissue Transplantation Research Panel, *Report,* 2.

62 T.H. Maugh, II, quoting Freed, "Doctor Who Broke Restriction on Fetal Tests Under Attack," *Los Angeles Times*, 21 November 1988, p. I3.

63 Lindvall, Rehncrona, Brundin, *et al.*, "Human Fetal Dopamine Neurons."

64 Human Fetal Tissue Transplantation Research Panel, *Report*, 29.

65 Robertson, "Fetal Tissue Transplants."

66 Human Fetal Tissue Transplantation Research Panel, *Report,* 2.

67 *Ibid.*, 4.

68 *Ibid.*

69 *Ibid.*, 6.

Part V

Use of Animals

Part V

Use of Animals

21

Evolving Ethical and Legal Norms in Animal Experimentation

T. David Marshall

I wish to propose that society, and more specifically the scientific community, approach this issue with a high degree of circumspection and prudence. There is no need to propose new ethical or philosophical principles too quickly, or to hastily impose restrictive legislation controlling the use of animals in medical research. New ethical or philosophical principles and restrictive legislation may be seen as the manifestation of a crisis or stampede mentality. This mentality may unduly restrict scientific freedom and impede important medical and social progress, because of premature acceptance of what may potentially be incorrect conclusions.

We should not be seeking some new advance in moral philosophy or ethics that would lead to a new code of rights for sentient animals used in research, or a new criminal code for research conduct to prevent abuse of animals in laboratories. Rather, we should be seeking an open and practical social method for establishing just and acceptable norms for the use of animals in research today.

I will first briefly explain what I consider to be "just" social norms. A *norm* may be described as a standard of conduct, or a right standard. If the norm is a just one, it is one that will be accepted as just by society, or at least by the dominant collective in society. In this sense, then, just norms are simply accepted norms.

Another feature of norms is that they are perpetually changing. In this century, changing norms in regard to the status of women and the nature of our sexual mores are ample evidence of this constant change.

Finally, like a hare before a pack of hounds, social norms are often followed by legislators and legislation. And it is not always possible to predict where these norms, like the hare, are likely to go. As in public policy, if one tries to put theory and principle ahead of the mature crystallization of public norms based on reality, the final reality of the norm will be something quite different from what the theorists predicted. Norms, in final form, are not easily prophesied; in fact, they seldom are. Recent moves to liberal democracy in Eastern Europe amply illustrate the failure of following theory that has not been proven or established empirically.

Just social norms, then, are difficult to divine, are a construct of society, and are ever changing. The question for us today is: How can we arrive at a just norm *pro tempore* in the use of experimental animals in medical research?

First, let us consider how society generally has sought these norms. In a democracy, these norms usually are based on what the people come to perceive as just under the current circumstances. Public representatives then convert these norms to public policy and perhaps legislation.

Norms are also place- and time-specific. One of the reasons we face a dilemma about the use of animals in research is that in many of its dimensions, it is a new concern. There are many reasons why this is so; I will cite just one, namely, that the majority of inhabitants of the Western world are no longer from an agricultural background. In my lifetime, in Canada, our society has changed from one that was predominantly rural to one that is predominantly urban.

The sincere outcry for legal and ethical protection for sentient animals in research, though not entirely new, has had a tremendous resurgence in the past decade. The common law as we know it developed in an agricultural society; as a result, there is no established legal matrix in common law to deal with this new and heightened sensitivity to animal suffering. The same could be said of our classic religious and philosophical configurations: an acceptance of animal use, though tempered with humanity, is a part of our religious and philosophic tradition. Therefore, there is little to guide us in quickly assimilating or changing the law or theory to accommodate what seem to the scientific community to be quite radical changes in our thinking. Indeed, the use of animals in research is a completely new paradigm in our culture. Before undertaking a radical transformation of the norms and policies upon which we have agreed for centuries, we must establish a process.

Therefore, in the use of animals in research today, we must all work to establish a process for arriving at just decisions and at new norms that will be seen by society as just. These will serve as empirical steps toward those new theories and new legislation that now elude us.

By creating such a process, we will indeed be working toward establishing new principles, and perhaps enacting new laws as well. However, what we need now is an acceptable process for moving forward. In the case of research with animals, what we seek is a process for dealing with a series of concrete cases. There are great variations in the levels of invasiveness in animal experimentation.

In addition, there are other variables such as the different levels of sentience in animal species. An infinite variety of scientific protocols could be imagined, each of which would raise a different degree of concern. Levels of social concern may also vary with time and place, and these variables must also be taken into account.

At this point, we do not need a mechanism for establishing general norms on a broad basis, such as a democratically elected legislature might provide. Nor do we require a more specific tool for establishing public policy like a royal commission or public inquiry. What we do need is a process that will seek acceptable (that is, just) norms, on a protocol by protocol (or case by case) basis.

There are two models that I wish to present that, in my opinion, may be seen as persuasive and illustrative metaphors. The first of these is the method used by common law courts to decide new situations not covered by earlier cases or established law. These so-called interstitial issues are not uncommon and, in the past, were the primary means of progress in the setting down of legal norms.

What I wish to emphasize is that the judge has no particular expertise in the subject matter of the litigation--indeed, it could be a social, scientific, architectural, or any other issue that requires a new norm. Regardless of that fact, the courts would have to establish a new norm *pro tempore*. Certain elements of this norm-finding process of the common law are of importance here.

First of all, the common law judge is, again, not an expert, but is reasonably intelligent and sensitive to his or her society. The judge is independent and impartial with regard to the resolution of the case before the court. The process is open and public. All conceivable arguments for and against the issue before the court are hopefully explored, as are the short- and long-term implications of a decision going one way or the other. This is now and has been historically an important societal method of establishing new norms.

I want to turn only briefly to a second paradigm, but this time from ethics. John Rawls, in an article entitled "Outline of a Decision Procedure for Ethics,"[1] describes a process similar to that used by the common law courts when they are faced with novel questions. Rawls's suggestion for novel questions involves the use not of experts in established or classical ethical theory, but rather of an eclectic group of reasonably intelligent people, fully briefed on all aspects of the problem--historic, social, and scientific--and on the possible ethical solutions. Here, too, the decisionmakers must be independent and impartial so as not to be compromised in decision making. Again, the process must be open to public input and public scrutiny.

It is interesting to note the parallels here. In novel situations in law, the judge, though learned in the law, has no real warrant by virtue of this legal knowledge to make new decisions. Nor do ethicists, in the process outlined by Rawls for novel ethical problems, have warrant by virtue of their knowledge to make new ethical decisions. They are essentially well-informed lay people.

The point is that, at base, both systems are really the same. In both systems, the decision makers are impartial, have a knowledge of all the facts and social repercussions, a lively intelligence, and sensitivity to the reality of our society. These qualities are some of the more important prerequisites for setting out novel, "just" norms.

I want to turn now specifically to the use of animals in research. What we seek in this case are just norms: that is, norms publicly seen as fair and acceptable norms. How do we arrive at them?

I believe we need a process or system that utilizes an eclectic, impartial group of intelligent and sensitive citizens fully versed in the reality of the situation--its social consequences and the various possible solutions in regard to the specific animal protocol under study.

I turn now to the Canadian experience as a paradigm in this regard. As in most jurisdictions, we have very basic legislation dealing with cruelty to animals.[2] In two provinces, we have legislation dealing with animals used in experimentation; again, this legislation sets out a very basic framework of control.

The cornerstone of our present system is what we call an Animal Research Ethics Board (AREB). The board, which is a committee established in each community, should be broadly based, with scientific members, lay members, and specialists in animal husbandry and the use of animals in research. We believe that the values of the community at large are essential to the work of the animal ethics board, and that it should contain not fewer than two members who have no direct relationship to the research community. They should bring community values to the deliberations.

Scientists with experience in research design are essential. We believe that research that is not scientifically valid is never justified. Animal care technicians who actually care for the research animals should be on the board to ensure that practical concerns are met.

We believe that a veterinarian specializing in laboratory animal medicine or appropriately trained to assess the invasiveness of the research is critical. To give the board a wide social base, bioethicists, philosophers, and social scientists are encouraged as members.

We are attempting now in Canada to implement not only uniform boards but uniform and open procedures. Issues such as length of approval, provisions for monitoring, and ongoing scrutiny are included. In Canada, the Canadian Council on Animal Care (CCAC)[3] oversees the functioning of the local committees (AREB). This body consists of a small secretariat and a number of veterinary surgeons experienced in the field of laboratory animals. The CCAC regularly visits institutions, reviews their procedures, and has the power to order improvements. The CCAC is funded by the agencies that provide grants to researchers and can suspend funding to those researchers who do not adhere to established regulations.

The process allows for appeals of decisions, effectively ensuring that *pro tempore* norms are always subject to change. If members of the AREB are seriously divided, other AREBs or the Canadian Council on Animal Care may be consulted. We have not proceeded with a national appeal board, preferring that the decision be made locally. If not accepted locally, then presumably the protocol should not go forward.

In summary, then, we should be concerned at this point entirely with process, rather than broad theory or legislation. This would be a process for decision making, no matter what that decision is--a process that is impartial, independent of research interests, well informed, representative, and, above all, open. This approach will ensure that evolving community norms are reflected in decisions, and that the community perceives these decisions as having been formulated in an open and just manner.

NOTES

1 J. Rawls, "Outline of a Decision Procedure for Ethics," in *Sources in Contemporary Philosophy: Ethics*, ed. J.J. Thomson and G. Dworkin (New York: Harper & Row, 1968), 55.
2 *Discussion Paper on the Use of Animals in Research* (Ottawa, ONT: Medical Research Council of Canada, October 1990).
3 *Guide to the Care and Use of Experimental Animals,* vol. 1 (Ottawa, ONT: Canadian Council on Animal Care, 1980); *Guide to the Care and Use of Experimental Animals,* vol. 2 (Ottawa, ONT: Canadian Council on Animal Care, 1984).

22

Protests about Animal Research and the Response from the Scientific and Medical Communities

M.J. Matfield

In this chapter I will review the use of animals in biological and medical research, and the protest that this research has engendered from some parts of the general public. I will highlight some of the motivations underlying this protest movement and discuss the ways in which the scientific and medical communities have responded to these protests.

Although the majority of the chapter focuses on the situation in Great Britain, whenever possible, I have made direct comparisons to the United States. There are great similarities between the situations in these two countries and for good reason: protestors from Great Britain have played an important part in stimulating the protest movement against animal research in the US.

Though its true that ancient Greek and Roman schools of medicine conducted some crude animal experimentation, animal research, as we now understand it, began in earnest with the scientific renaissance of the 17th century.[1] Francis Bacon's concept of experimental science was applied by a number of early biologists who discovered many of the fundamental principals of mammalian biology in the decades that followed (see Table 22.1). This new science of experimental physiology continued into the 18th and 19th century with the first measurement of blood pressure, the establishment of experimental surgery, and the discovery of spinal reflexes by Marshall Hall: all of which depended on the use of animals in research.

Although animal experiments were the subject of occasional criticisms in learned essays during the late 18th and early 19th century, it was not until the middle of the 19th century that antivivisection protests truly became established. In 1863, Frances Power Cobbe, an English journalist, was responsible for

TABLE 22.1

Early Examples of Animal Experimentation, Showing the Tremendous Effect of Bacon's Experimental Method upon Animal Research

YEAR	DISCOVERY
500 BC-200 AD	Aristotelian and Hippocratic experimental studies
1540	Early Atomists
1620	Francis Bacon: Principles of experimental science
1627	Aselli: Discovery of the lymphatic system
1628	Harvey: Discovery of blood circulation
1661	Malpighi: Discovery of capillaries
1667	Hooke: Discovery of the function of lungs

initiating the world's first organized antivivisection protest.[2] When travelling in Italy, she became acquainted with the animal research of Professor Moritz Schiff in Florence and organized a petition against his work amongst the local nobility and English expatriate community. On returning to Britain, Cobbe continued her campaigning and founded the world's first antivivisection organization, the Victoria Street Society. She set about recruiting support amongst members of parliament, resulting in the first proposal for legislation to ban animal experiments. A debate amongst members of parliament followed, leading to the formation of a Royal Commission of Inquiry.[3] This, in turn, led to the government proposing legislation to control animal experiments in 1876. The first draft of this legislation, written by the supporters of Cobbe, was extremely restrictive. The scientific and medical communities responded by energetically lobbying members of Parliament.[4] A short but intense struggle ensued, which ended in victory for the scientific lobby and the substantial moderation of the provisions of the bill before it was passed as legislation.[5]

The antivivisection movement, believing they had been betrayed, set about organizing a substantial campaign to swing public opinion against animal experimentation. Thus was born the great antivivisection movement of the late Victorian period in Britain. It involved many notable figures in society with numerous books, articles, public lectures, and meetings devoted to the denouncement of animal experimenters and their research.

In the US, protest about animal research followed a similar course. The American Antivivisection Society was founded in 1883 by Caroline Earl White, a woman who greatly admired and was heavily influenced by Frances Power Cobbe and her campaigning in Britain.[6] Although there was not nearly as much protest about animal research in the US during this period, the course of events was quite similar to that in Britain. In both countries, many antivivisection societies were formed, which were dominated by middle-class ladies who actively recruited support amongst members of their legislature and medical community. The medical and scientific communities in both countries responded, organizing themselves to lobby against proposals for restrictive legislation, as well as educating their own colleagues of the value of animal research. In Great Britain, the Physiological Society (1876), the Association for the Advancement of Medicine by Research (1882), and the Research Defense Society (1908) were founded for this purpose. In the US, the American Medical Association founded the Council for the Defense of Medical Research in 1907. The public education efforts of these organizations, combined with the effect of the First World War and the subsequent social changes, more or less completely dissipated the antivivisection protest movement of the period.

This history is illustrated by the crude measure of enumerating antivivisection books published in each of the two countries.[7] Figure 22.1 shows how antivivisection sentiment originated in Britain and Europe, developing into a significant protest movement by the end of the 19th century. The protest movement in the US started about twenty years later, in many ways stimulated by the British protest movement, but it never reached the magnitude of its UK counterpart. This graph also clearly shows how protest about animal experiments has grown massively over the last thirty years. Whereas the antivivisection

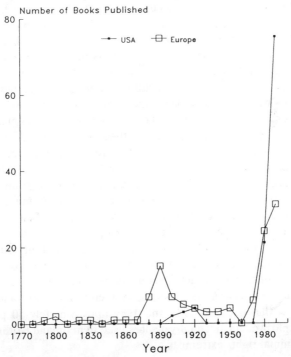

Fig. 22.1. Ten-year totals of the numbers of books objecting to animal experimentation published in the US and Europe.

protests at the beginning of this century were stimulated by anger about the real and imagined suffering involved for laboratory animals, the wellspring of present-day protest is a philosophical concept: the idea of animal rights.

A slightly more sophisticated analysis of the information, featured in the last few decades of this graph, shows how the concept of animal rights has developed.[8] Figure 22.2 gives the number of books published in each five-year period in Europe that either argue for animal rights in general, or specifically against animal research. The vast majority of these are British publications. It can be seen that the animal rights publications start earlier and, apart from a drop in the late 1960s, their rate of publication grows more rapidly than the books that are specifically against animal research. This illustrates that, over the last thirty years, sentiment against animal research has been a product of the animal rights philosophy. A similar analysis for the US (Figure 22.3) shows the same effect; animal rights publications proceeded, and were more numerous than, publications against animal research. However, it is noticeable that these trends began later in the US, but rise much more rapidly, ultimately resulting in far more books of both types published in the US than in Britain over the last twenty years.

Philosophical questioning about whether animals had intrinsic rights started with Jeremy Bentham in 1780 but, until relatively recently, it remained a somewhat obscure point of view with no popular support. It was revived in 1965 by the writer Bridget Brophy in an essay published in a major British national newspaper.[9] During the late 1960s and 1970s the idea of animal rights gave birth to a entire campaign movement in Great Britain. This was fueled, at one end, by a group of young philosophers and writers at Oxford University, including Peter Singer and Richard Ryder, two acknowledged father figures of the modern animal rights movement.[10] Their writings influenced a number of American philosophers who embraced the animal rights concepts with considerable fervor. Foremost amongst these is Tom Regan, whose 1983 magnum opus, *A Case For Animal Rights*,[11] is still probably the most substantial book arguing this case. At the other end of the spectrum, the animal rights movement was fed by a growing extremism. In 1974, the Band of Mercy was founded by the anti-hunting activist Ronnie Lee. This group carried out the first animal liberation raids on university animal houses and arson attacks on pharmaceutical research facilities.[12] After serving a jail sentence for arson attacks, Ronnie Lee renamed his organization the Animal Liberation Front (or ALF). From these beginnings in the United Kingdom, ALF has spread to over twenty-four countries and has been responsible, mostly in Britain, for numerous thefts of animals from research facilities, arson attacks, letter bombs, and the use of anti-personnel explosive devices, as well as countless incidents of minor vandalism. Police figures show that between 1985 and 1989 approximately 50 percent of the terrorist explosive and incendiary devices used in mainland Britain were attributable to animal rights extremists.

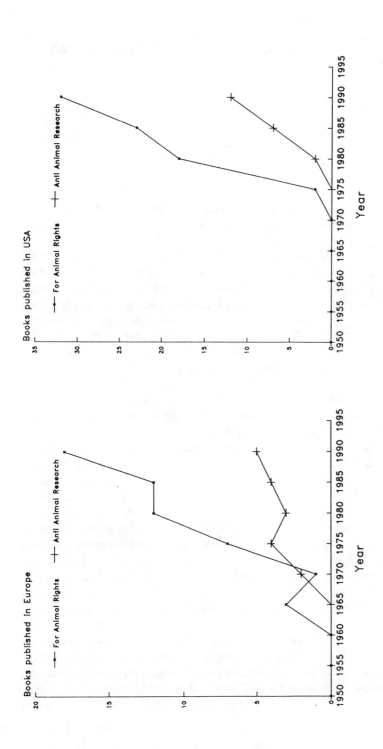

Fig. 22.2. Five-year totals of the numbers of books published that either argue for animal rights or against animal research in Europe.

Fig. 22.3. Five-year totals of the numbers of books published that either argue for animal rights or against animal research in the US.

TABLE 22.2

Figures from the Annual Reports and Accounts of 1989 of the British Union for the Abolition of Vivisection, National Antivivisection Society and Annual Aid

NAME	MEMBERSHIP	INCOME P.A.
BUAC	16,000	£1,100,00
NAVS	9,000	£960,000
Animal Aid	18,000	£530,000

The philosophy of animal rights holds that all sentient beings share the same intrinsic rights, and human beings have no special rights to themselves. From this premise, the philosophy of animal rights argues that any use of animals by humans is immoral or unethical. Bias toward our own species is thus termed *speciesism* and is regarded as the equivalent of racism or slavery.[13] It is important to distinguish between the idea of animal rights and animal welfare. Animal welfare, the acceptance of a duty to care for animals in our charge, preventing cruelty or unnecessary suffering to them, is a majority view in most Western countries. The concept of animal rights, which fundamentally opposes all use of animals--for human entertainment, sport, or companionship, in agriculture and research--is clearly a minority point of view that runs counter to the practices of most Western societies.

In Britain, there are three major animal rights organizations: the British Union of the Abolition of Vivisection (BUAV), the National Anti-Vivisection Society (NAVS) and Animal Aid (Table 22.2). BUAV and NAVS started as active antivivisection organizations during the heyday of late Victorian antivivisection protest. They were inactive and moribund by the 1970s, until they were taken over and radicalized by animal rights activists. Entryism and radicalization was also attempted on the RSPCA--the oldest and most respected animal welfare charity--but this did not succeed.[14] Animal Aid is a more recent organization, founded in 1977, but it has had a remarkable growth in recent years. Figures for 1989 give these three animal rights organizations a combined membership of 43,000 and a combined income of approximately £2.5 million per annum. By comparison, in the US there is one dominate animal rights organization, People for the Ethical Treatment of Animals (PETA). It was founded in 1980 and, in 1986, one of the leading British animal rights activists, Kim Stallwood, moved to the US to become the Executive Director of PETA,[15] helping it achieve its current size of nearly 300,000 members with an annual income of over $6 million.[16] In the US there has also been a growing radicalization of the old established humane and animal protection organizations, the Humane Society of the United States and the American Society of the Prevention of Cruelty to Animals. These organizations, with their very substantial membership and funding, have been viewed as prime targets for entryism by animal rights activists.

The campaigning tactics of animal rights organizations on both sides of the Atlantic are similar, but there is significantly more violence and extremism in Great Britain. The use of overblown and distorted propaganda is common to both, as is the tactic of targeting individual researchers with demonstrations, adverse publicity, harassment, intimidation, and death threats. The claim that animal experimentation causes medical harm, either by creating new diseases or being responsible for massive harmful drug side effects, is frequently aired.[17]

The very active campaigning directed at children by the animal rights organizations is of particular concern.[18] In Britain, the British Union for the Abolition of Vivisection has a number of campaign buses that carry a mobile exhibition aimed at school children, with the buses stopping each day at a new school. The appeal of the animal rights message to adolescents should not be underestimated. Not only is it radical and anti-establishment, with a clear role for individual involvement, but it can also be portrayed as very good--as being "green" and as being nice to animals. Other, more dubious tactics found on both sides of the Atlantic include the deliberate infiltration of animal research facilities by animal rights activists who take jobs as technicians or cleaners. Whilst the initial publicity given to the "exposé" by the infiltrator may not seem too serious, these are usually accompanied by demonstrations, intimidation, and threats against the research directors and their families, and real or faked bomb threats.[19] The documents removed by the infiltrator can be used to cause commercial damage, and can lead to lengthy legal wrangles, wasting large amounts of private and public money.[20]

Outright terrorist activities by the animal rights movements are far more frequent in Great Britain than any other country. The firebombing of department stores that sell fur coats has been a favorite tactic since 1985.[21] In most cases, the incendiary devices start a small blaze that triggers the sprinkler system, ruining the entire stock and damaging the flooring and decoration of the building. However, in some cases, incendiary devices have been planted in stores where the sprinkler system was not functioning, with significantly greater damage ensuing. The arson of the Dingles department store in Plymouth in 1989 is probably the largest single act of domestic terrorism in financial terms that has ever occurred in Great Britain. The entire building was gutted, with substantial damage to adjacent buildings and loss of trade for over two years. The consequential loss to the company was said to be in excess of £180 million.

The car bomb has been used on nearly thrity occasions by animal rights extremists in Great Britain. Many of the early car bomb devices were very crude in construction, frequently failed to explode, and appeared designed to destroy the parked car rather than to kill anyone attempting to drive it. However, the bombers grew more sophisticated and gradually produced more dangerous devices. The two most recent car bombings in Britain have used high-explosive devices triggered by a mercury tilt switch when the car begins to move. In their style of construction and deployment, these devices were clearly designed to kill the two animal researchers under whose cars they were placed. It was only by a combination of extreme good fortune and very prompt action that both individuals escaped with only minor injuries. Tragically, in one case, a passerby was seriously injured.[22]

Despite intensive police investigation, no one has been charged with these crimes. Although the police were not able to determine the identities of those responsible for the bombings, evidence was found to suggest that the bombers had a plentiful supply of high explosives, and that there was every indication that they would strike again. The increasing sophistication of these attacks makes it quite probable that the next victims will be killed. Everyone working with, or connected to, animal research in Britain today is advised by the police to check under their vehicle before they use it.

The response of the medical and scientific communities to the animal rights campaigning against animal experimentation has included both legislative lobbying and public education. In both Britain and the US, new legislation to control animal research has been implemented. Although the extreme animal rights organizations have played little part in these legislative initiatives, there was considerable lobbying on both sides of the Atlantic by more moderate animal-protection organizations and by scientific and medical organizations over the details of the legislation.

The main thrust of the public education efforts have focused on informing the public about the benefits of animal research. A great number of the major medical advances of the last century have depended on animal research (Table 22.3).[23] It is noticeable that the response by the medical and scientific communities in America has been much more energetic than that in Britain. Organizations representing the scientific and clinical communities, such as the Foundation for Biomedical Research and patient organizations, such as Incurably Ill for Medical Research, have produced a substantial volume of well-designed and effective literature concerning the use of animals in biomedical research and testing. More recently, some of these organizations have produced some eye-catching and arresting posters to promote the understanding of the general public.

Scientific and medical spokesmen have been trained in the most effective techniques for communicating their point of view on television and radio--both of which play important roles in influencing the views of the general public. Indeed, the media themselves are often in need of education about the subject of animal experimentation and, in Britain, we have found that a most effective way of providing information is through a "Declaration on Animals in Medical Research."[24] This declaration was drafted by the British Association for the Advancement of Science, well known to the media as the most prestigious voice

TABLE 22.3

Major Medical Advances that Depended on Animal Research

YEAR	ADVANCE
1920s	Insulin for diabeties
1930s	Modern anaesthetics for surgery
	Diptheria vaccine
1940s	Broad-spectrum antibiotics for infections
	Whoolping couch vaccine
	Heart-lung machine for open-heart surgery
1950s	Kidney transplants
	Cardiac pagemakers and replacement heart valves
	Polio vaccine
	Drugs for high blood pressure
	Hip replacement surgery
1960s	Corneal transplants
	Rubella vaccine
	Coronary bypass operation
	Heart transplants
	Drugs to treat mental illness
1970s	Drugs to treat ulcers
	Improved sututures and other surgical techniques
	Drugs to treat asthma
	Drugs to treat leukimia
1980s	Immunosuppressant drugs for organ transplants
	CAT scanning for improve diagnosis
	Life-support sustens for premature babies
	Drugs to treat virus disease

of British science. The declaration states, in simple terms, the importance of animal research both for past medical advances and for future research into killer diseases. It also emphasizes the importance of high standards for the welfare of laboratory animals and the need for informed and sensible public discussion of the issues involved.

Over the last eight or nine months this declaration has been signed by nearly 1,000 professors of medicine and biomedical scientists, as well as leading clinicians and researchers, and representatives from many medical and scientific research organizations. Faced with such a clear statement, with such overwhelming, eminent medical and scientific support, many journalists are willing to trust the points made in the declaration.

We have to realize that the medical and scientific communities will always be at a disadvantage in trying to inform the public about animal research. It is in the very nature of news reporting to have a substantial bias against the status quo. In simple terms, saying that the status quo is all right is not news and will not get reported. However, a statement that says the status quo is wrong will be, by definition, newsworthy and far more likely to get reported. While there have been countless newspaper articles criticizing animal research, the number stating the medical and scientific case for careful, humane, and properly controlled animal research are far fewer. However, the efforts of organizations like the Foundation for Biomedical Research and the Research Defense Society have ensured that our point of view is put across to the public in the newspapers and television. By continuing these efforts, we hope to be able to balance the increasingly strident views expressed by the animal rights movement.

NOTES

1   R.D. French, *Antivivisection and Medical Science in Victorian Society* (Princeton: Princeton University Press, 1975).
2   F.D. Cobbe, *Life of Frances Power Cobbe* (London, 1894).
3   *Report of the Royal Commission on the Practice of Subjecting Live Animals to Experiments for Scientific Purposes* (London: Her Majesty's Stationery Office, (HMSO), 1876).
4   French, *Antivivisection*.
5   *Cruelty to Animals Act* (London: Her Majesty's Stationery Office (HMSO), 1876).
6   S.E. Lederer, "The Controversy over Animal Experiments in America, 1880-1914," in N.A. Rupke, *Vivisection in Historical Perspective* (Kent: Croon Helm, 1987), 236-258.
7   French, *Antivivisection*; C.R. Magel, *Keyguide to Information Sources in Animal Rights* (London: Mansell Publishing, 1989); N.A. Rupke, *Vivisection in Historical Perspective* (Kent: Croon Helm, 1987).
8   Magel, *Keyguide to Information*.
9   B. Brophy, "The Rights of Animals," (London) *Sunday Times*, 10 October 1965.
10   R.D. Ryder, *Animal Revolution* (Oxford, England: Basil Blackwell, 1989).
11   T. Regan, *The Case for Animal Rights* (Berkley: University of California Press, 1983).
12   D. Henshaw, *Animal Warfare: The Story of the Animal Liberation Front* (London: Fontana, 1989).
13   P. Singer, *Animal Liberation*, 2nd ed. (London: Johnathan Cape, 1990).
14   Henshaw, *Animal Warfare*.
15   *Ibid.*

16 *Directory of Animal Rights/Welfare Organizations* (Washington, DC: Foundation for Biomedical Research, 1990).

17 *Biohazard* (London: National Anti-Vivisection Society, 1987); *Health with Humanity* (London: British Union for the Abolition of Vivisection, 1990).

18 H. Sutton, "Animal Lobby Tries Kid Stuff," *PR Week* (8 March 1990).

19 "Huntingdon Research Centre," *RDS Newsletter* (publication of the Research Defence Society, London), (July 1990).

20 K. McCabe, "Beyond Cruelty," *The Washingtonian*, 25, no.5 (February 1990).

21 Henshaw, *Animal Warfare*.

22 M. Matfield, "The Return of the Bombers," *RDS Newsletter* (July 1990).

23 W. Paton, "Man and Mouse," in *Animals in Medical Research* (Oxford: Oxford University Press, 1984).

24 "British Association Declares Support for Animal Research," *RDS Newsletter* (October 1990).